Slaughter and Preservation of Meat

by

SANDOL JOHNSON, PhD

Illustrations by
BETH ROBINSON, DVM

Cover by
TODD COONEY, DVM

Christian Veterinary Mission

A Publication of Christian Veterinary Mission

Christian Veterinary Mission
19303 Fremont Avenue North
Seattle, WA 98133 USA
Current Book Information at:
www.cvmusa.org
PHONE: (206) 546-7569 FAX: (206) 546-7458

Library of Congress Cataloging-in-Publication Data

Johnson, Sandol.
Slaughter and preservation of meat / by Sandol Johnson ; illustrations by Beth Robinson ; cover by Todd Cooney.
p. cm.—(Raising healthy animals series)
Includes bibliographical references and index.
ISBN 1-886532-16-8
1. Meat—Preservation. I. Title. II. Series.
TS1960.J6 2005
664'.9—dc22

2005010607

Raising Healthy Animals Series

Every year, thousands of people around the world struggle to survive because they don't have the right knowledge, skills and resources to care for their animals. Christian Veterinary Mission (CVM) sends veterinary professionals to live and work alongside many of these people to encourage them and provide them with not only much needed veterinary expertise, but also the hope that is only found in Christ. CVM veterinarians build lasting relationships with individuals and communities, helping them be transformed through Christ's love.

CVM, in its effort to be meaningfully involved in work in the developing world, quickly found there was little appropriate educational material available. CVM set about developing basic resource materials in animal husbandry for farmers and agricultural workers. Apparently, they met a real need, as these books have been accepted throughout the developing nations of the world.

The series of books published by Christian Veterinary Mission includes the following in order of publication:

Raising Healthy Pigs *	Drugs and Their Usage
Raising Healthy Rabbits *	Where There Is No Animal Doctor
Raising Healthy Fish	Raising Healthy Horses
Raising Healthy Cattle	Zoonoses: Animal Diseases That Affect Humans
Raising Healthy Poultry *+	Raising Healthy Honey Bees
Raising Healthy Goats *	Slaughter and Preservation of Meat
Raising Healthy Sheep	Disease and Parasite Prevention in Farm Animals

[Also available in: * Spanish + French].

CVM fieldworkers have also developed specific training materials for the countries in which they work.

All of these books have been put together by Christian men and women; in a labor of love and service, for people in need throughout the world. It demonstrates dedication to their profession, service to humanity and a witness to their faith. We hope that they are a help to you in developing an appropriate livestock program to meet your needs. We pray God's blessing on their use.

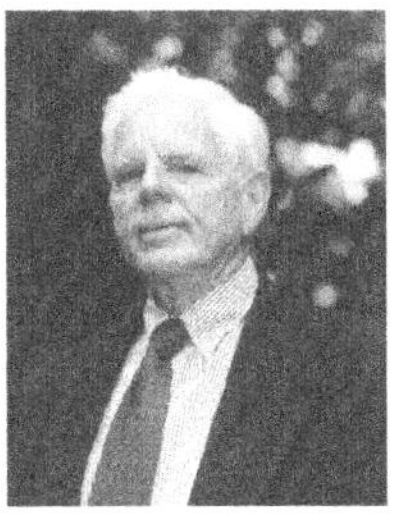

Leroy Dorminy
CVM Founder

Dedication

This book has been a labor of love more than time. I wish to dedicate this book to the late, Ronald E. (Skip) Engel; the original author. Though, he was unable to complete this book, I became aware of his dedication to this project through his research files that I received. Dr. Engel was an enthusiastic supporter of this project and was giving his whole heart, unfortunately, he was not able to finish this mission.

I truly am grateful to Dr. Leroy Dorminy, founder of CVM, for giving me the honor of completing this work that Dr. Engel began. Dr. Dorminy has offered only encouragement and unshakeable confidence that the book would be completed. I have learned perseverance and humbleness from Dr. Dorminy through this work.

I would also like to dedicate this book to Dr. Earle Goodman, who reread many manuscripts and gave detailed corrections. He has worked tirelessly in the Healthy Animal Series as an editor for many other books as well.

This book is also dedicated to Dr. Ted Montgomery, my first meat science professor in college, who has expressed only support in my endeavors; and Dr. Ruth Blackburn, USDA Veterinarian in Charge, who taught me many aspects of pathology in the slaughter plant.

Also, I dedicate this book to my family: my late parents, Vernon and Frances Johnson; and my late husband, Darrell Gwartney; who always supported my animal science career. Special thanks to my son, Micah, who signed me up with the CVM many years ago and who has been enthusiastic about this project.

I also dedicate this to the many ministers in my life who have prayed for me and helped me to come to know Jesus Christ.

PSALMS 139:13-14

For Thou (God) didst form my inward parts; Thou didst weave me in my mother's womb. I will give thanks to Thee, for I am fearfully and wonderfully made; Wonderful are Thy (God) works, and my soul knows it very well.

Table of Contents

Section I

Background and Introduction

BACKGROUND

This book is made available by Christian Veterinary Missions to provide basic information concerning slaughter, processing and preserving meat for missionaries, small farmers, and agricultural workers. The topics discussed are Sanitation, Pre-slaughter (Ante-mortem) conditions, and Post-slaughter (Post-mortem) conditions with abnormalities, Beef Slaughter and Processing, Sheep Slaughter and Processing, Poultry Slaughter and Processing, Small Animal Slaughter and Processing, Preservation, Storage, Simple Slaughter Facility, and Small to Medium Plant Plans.

The last section of this book discusses the small to medium size slaughter and processing facilities. This should be utilized as a reference for people that continue to expand the number of animals they slaughter and process.

INTRODUCTION

All countries have animals that are raised as a source of nutrition. It may be an individually raised animal or a small herd that meets the need of meat protein for the people. With this comes a means of slaughter. The proper sanitation, as well as, the proper inspection of the animal and its meat is provided in this book to prevent spread of diseases to humans.

We recognize that there are many cultures and traditions that utilize various animals and animal products. There are many that are not utilized by certain cultures. However, this book was written to be a guide for a variety of animals and their usage and it is not intended to be either an endorsement or an aversion.

This book is intended to assist the small farmer, missionary, or agricultural worker in the proper methods of slaughter of meat animals and in the preservation of the meat products. The proper methods for preparation of meat for human consumption are important to maintain proper human health.

Section II

Sanitation and Cleanliness

Chapter 1

Cleanliness of Facility, Hand Washing and Personal Hygiene, Cleaning Knives and Equipment

Cleanliness of the Facility

I PETER 4:10

As each one has received a special gift, employ it in serving one another, as good stewards of the manifold grace of God.

Why the Facility Should be Kept Clean

Pests (vermin)

1. The area that will be used to slaughter should be clean and free from trash. If working outside on a cement slab, that area shall still be very clean and kept as dry as possible.

2. Trash or items stacked up will bring in rats and mice. Rats, mice, cats, dogs, insects, birds, and lizards all can be called a pest (vermin). A pest will be around a slaughter area and try to find and carry off parts of an animal for food.

3. Insects will fly and land on the animals, carcasses, and meat parts to pick up food.

4. Flies live around the latrine, livestock or areas of trash and then fly into areas of slaughter and processing. The flies will get on the carcass and meat products and leave the disease they are carrying on the meat. Flies lay their eggs on trash and food particles. These eggs will hatch and bring in more flies.

5. Pests (vermin) like to live in trash and around places where there is food to eat. Rats and mice will move into these areas. They carry disease with their droppings. They will accumulate outside of an area and try to come inside the facility.

6. Wandering animals such as cats and dogs can be hard pests to run off. Dogs should not be allowed anywhere near areas of slaughter or processing. Dogs may also carry diseases and filth. Dogs will try to lap up blood and take pieces of the carcass off. This should not be allowed. This can spread disease from diseased animals to humans.

7. Cats will climb and move around areas where dogs cannot get to. If at all possible cats should not be allowed in areas of slaughter and processing.

8. Lizards also climb up over roofs and around buildings. Their droppings can also carry diseases.

9. Birds can do much damage by roosting in roofs and in trees surrounding the slaughter and processing area. The droppings and feathers are not wanted around areas of meat processing.

10. Other livestock and animals should not be roaming free around the areas of slaughter and processing. Other animals could be carrying diseases or filth that could come in contact with the live animal before slaughter and the carcass and meat products after slaughter.

11. If possible, flies must be kept out with screens on windows and doors, or a fly fan over doors.

12. Moving waste away from areas of slaughter and meat processing will keep pests from living in the trash and waste. A designated area away from the slaughter facility should be found.

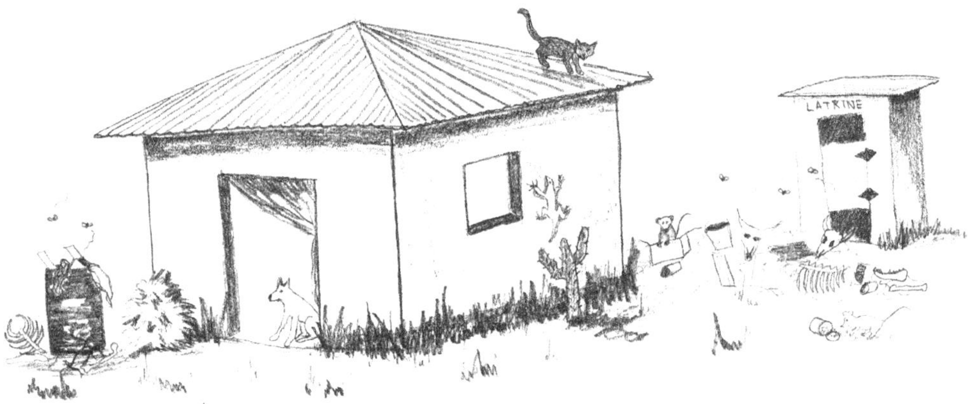

A Bad Facility—vermin, trash, latrine close by, grass growing up, no door, no window coverings.

Germs (microorganisms)

1. Dirt, mud, hair, blood, dried fat, meat particles, standing water, dirty water, and dirty equipment are all areas that allow flies and pests (vermin) to live. There are also germs (microorganisms) that can begin to grow very rapidly in the same areas.

6. The germs (microorganisms) cannot be seen by the human eye. They may be called bacteria and are what cause disease in animals and humans.

7. The microorganisms may even be in a resting period or dormant period until there is a food (nutrient) available for them to feed on to begin to grow. Germs (microorganisms) are like people they need air, water, normal temperature, and a food supply to grow. All of this is found in and around a place of slaughter and processing.

8. When the microorganism comes in contact with a meat or meat product, they can become attached to the meat and then begin to grow very quickly. Meat and meat products provide a very good source for the microorganisms to grow.

10. This is why all parts of the facility should be cleaned after each day's work. If it is very dirty, clean or rinse down between animals that are slaughtered and processed.

Processes to Keep a Clean Facility

1. Water is the most important way to keep a facility and workers clean. The area should be rinsed with water as hot as possible (70° C; 160° F).

2. If a food grade detergent is available, it should be used next with water. The detergent can be added to a bucket of water to use for scrubbing with a scrub brush. The water should be soapy and a scrub brush used to scrub all areas and equipment.

3. Wash the detergent off with hot water; leave no soap. Water with chlorinated bleach (Clorox) should be used if hot water is not available and used as a final sanitizer. Cleaning after slaughter or processing with hot water will get rid of blood and fat that can dry on work areas and give a place for microorganisms to grow.

4. To begin working, the area should be checked for cleanliness. Just asking basic questions will help find areas that need to be cleaned before a new day of working.

a. Did it get cleaned before this use?
b. Is there any trash that needs to be moved?
c. Is there any dried blood or fat on floors, equipment or tables?
d. Is there any hair from a previous animal's slaughter?
e. Is all equipment clean?
f. Are the floors and walls clean?
g. Are the workers clean?
h. Are the workers' clothing and body clean?
i. Are the holding facilities for the live animals clean with fresh water for the animals to drink?
j. Is the processing area clean?
k. Are all storage areas clean and free from blood and water?

5. The areas that the live animal, carcass, meat and meat products come in contact with are all potentially dangerous to pick up disease from un-cleanliness. This is very important not only for human's health, but also to keep the meat and meat products from spoiling.

6. Microorganisms work as a spoilage factor in meat and meat products. They will cause meat to spoil quickly. Even when meat is processed and preserved with spices there may still be microorganisms on the meat that can cause diseases.

Separation of lavatories and work areas

1. Toilet rooms should be properly ventilated and should be separated from exposed product rooms by either a vestibule or a dressing room.

2. If modern plumbing is not available, the outside toilet should be some distance away from the facility.

3. Always wash hands after going to the latrine (toilet). Use fresh running water and soap, if available.

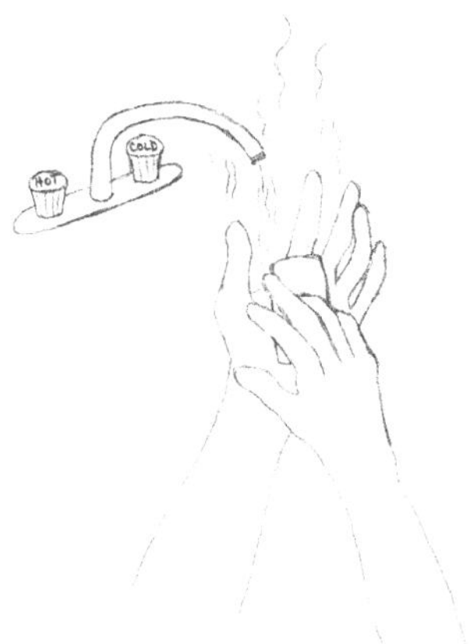

Wash hands with soap and water.

Storage Areas of the Facility

1. Dry storage of non-food material should be in a dry area away from slaughter and processing areas.

2. Detergents, disinfectants and similar substances should be stored separately from food and from wrapping and packaging material.

Separate storage of edible and inedible products

1. Condemned and other inedible (not for human food) meat and offal (internal organs) should be removed in a hygienic manner, and as quickly as possible, from rooms containing edible material.

2. The condemned meat and the inedible parts should be disposed of by digging a hole, covering the condemned meat and parts with lime and covering it with soil. Condemned meat should not be fed to dogs.

3. Offal should be removed immediately after slaughter to an area away from the clean carcass. Offal can be opened and the ingesta (food part) removed and dumped in a separate area or barrel away from the facility. The offal should be divided and cleaned inside and outside, if kept for human food. It is important that it is thoroughly cleaned of any ingesta (food part), and rinsed continually in cool water until it is clean.

4. Offal not to be kept for human food should be emptied of the ingesta and boiled down before it is given to any animal for food. The boiling will kill any parasites that may be in the offal.

5. If offal is to be stored, it should be kept cool and separate from meat from the carcass until later use.

6. Hides should be removed to a separate area inside or outside of the facility that is only for hides. This prevents cross contamination of the dirt and hair on the hides with the carcass and meat products. The hides can then be further cleaned and made ready for tanning if in a separate area.

Requirements for walls and floor junctions

1. Walls should be smooth, durable, impermeable, and of a color which permits detection of unsanitary conditions. White wash with lime is common.

2. Walls should have washable surfaces.

3. Walls and floor junctions should be constructed and maintained so as to assure that surfaces are clean and free of contamination.

4. A molding that will connect the floor to the wall should be used that makes cleaning easier. If this is not possible a sealant for the cracks between walls and floors will help maintain sanitary conditions.

Waste water

1. The facility should have a drainage and plumbing system that is effective.

2. All the drains and gutters should be properly installed with traps, vents, or screens to collect excess fat, pieces of meat, hair and other large debris.

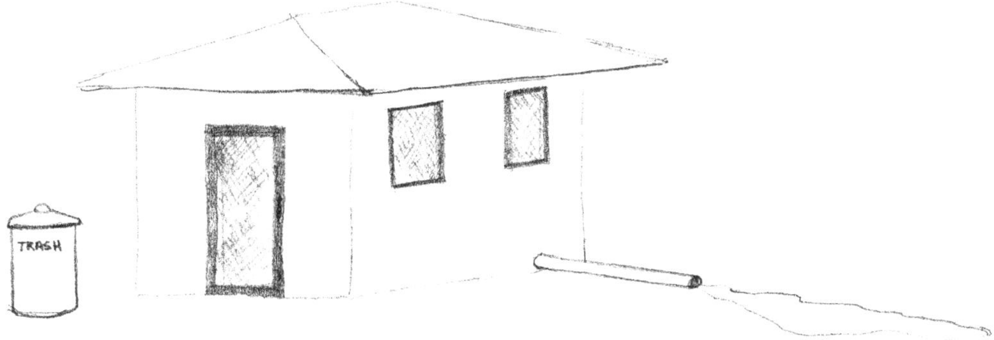

This is a clean facility, it has a door and window coverings. There is a pipe to drain outside of the building and trash kept outside of the building.

Structural wood

1. Wooden structures should be in good condition, impermeable, smooth, durable, rot-proof and sealed with a waterproof coating.

Roofs

1. Roofs should be made of a material that protects the slaughter area from rain, dirt, birds, vermin, and anything from falling or coming inside the slaughter or processing area. Materials will vary in different regions.

2. Roofs should be over the simple slaughter facility (that may only be a concrete floor) and over the more advanced facilities.

Hand washing Equipment

1. A sink should be made available for workers to wash their hands. Running cold and hot water with soap should be made available for workers before they begin work and at intervals during the day.

2. Hand wash basins in processing rooms and lavatories must not be hand-operated, they must be foot operated, if possible.

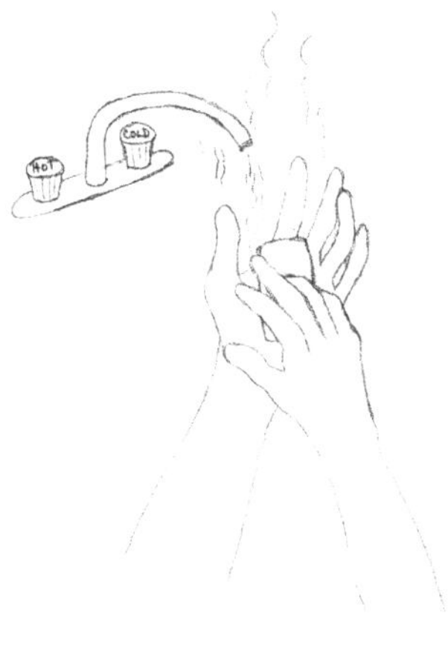

Hand wash sinks should be foot operated, if possible.

Sterilization of utensils and implements

1. Facilities should provide boiling water (sanitizing) to clean knives and equipment as often as necessary. Implements such as knives or hooks which come into contact with meat should be cleaned and boiled (sanitized) many times during the day.

2. When knives and hooks come in contact with contaminated material or surfaces such as the external surfaces of hides, boiling (sanitizing) should be completed. Sanitization should be done with 70° C or hotter (160° F or hotter) water.

3. Knives previously used in slaughter process should be cleaned and boiled (sanitized) before use in further processing. Chlorinated (Clorox) bleach should be used after scrubbing and rinsing the knives for better sanitizing.

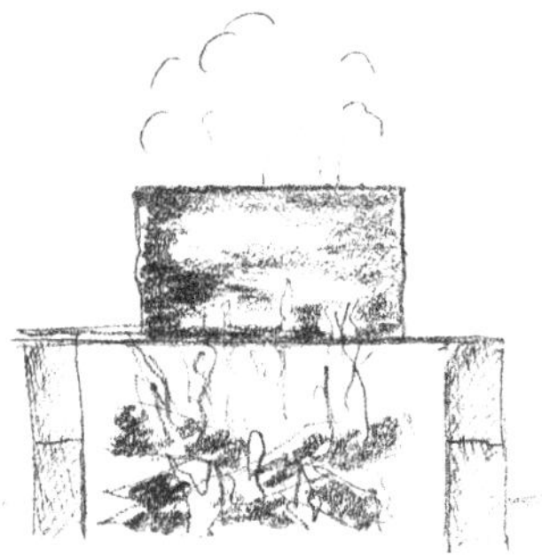

Clean with hot water.

Employee Health

1. Workers in the facility that come in direct contact with meat and meat products should be in good health and have no open sores on the hands or arms.

2. The facility should have a program to monitor employee health, by a health care person.

3. All cases of suspected diseases should be referred to a medical doctor for diagnosis.

4. Facilities shall keep records of medical examinations.

5. The above items (guidelines) for Employee Health may not be possible at any given time. It is advisable to follow all guidelines that can be done.

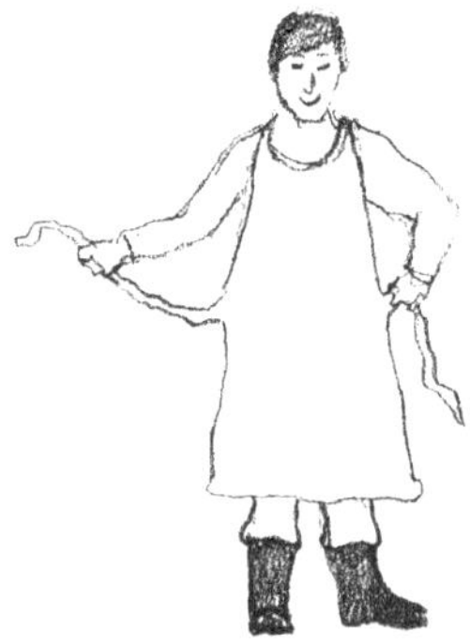

Employees (workers) should be in good health and have no open sores.

Hand Washing and Personal Hygiene

Upon arrival for work, the processor should wash their hands and arms up to their elbows with soap and warm water. Whatever was on the hands and arms of the worker can be transferred to the carcass and meat products they are working with.

The hands and arms should be scrubbed with soap, warm water and rinsed and dried with a clean towel or disposable towels. Clean towels prevent the spread of bacteria.

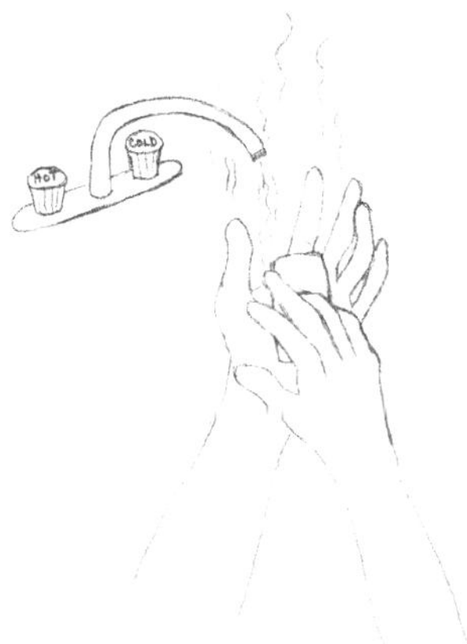

Wash hands often when working with the carcass.

Hands should be rewashed after coming in contact with outside part of a carcass. The outside part of the carcass may have dirt, fecal material, and other undesirable germs (microorganisms) on the hair, hide or skin that could be passed onto the clean fat and meat portion of the carcass.

Clean clothing should be worn each new day of processing. Clothing that has been worn before (dirty) will contain germs (bacteria). These germs could come in contact with meat products and begin to grow very quickly.

Clothing that has blood spots should be soaked in salty water or a degreaser to loosen the blood. The clothing may be washed first in cold water and salt or when all the blood is removed in warm water with a good detergent.

Human hair like that of the animal may contain bacteria and dirt. Hair should be kept up in a hairnet, clean cap or a hard hat if overhead objects will be used. Hair can fall onto the carcass and meat that is being cut up. Anything on the hair will then be left on the carcass or meat, even after the hair is picked off the carcass or meat. Hair should not be allowed to get onto the meat or meat product.

The worker's hair and body should be clean.

Jewelry should not be worn, because it could fall into a meat product and be found later in the meat or in someone's mouth. Jewelry also hinders some processors' working ability and irritations from blood, water and soap could occur.

The key to having good sanitation begins with the workers and their equipment. Workers' clothing and work equipment should all be washable and able to withstand warm to hot water.

Equipment should be washed between animals and between slaughter and processing areas. This prevents any contamination or disease being transferred from one animal or animal part to another animal or animal part.

The equipment should be hosed down with warm to hot water 70° C (160 ° F) and if there is excess grime, should be scrubbed with soap.

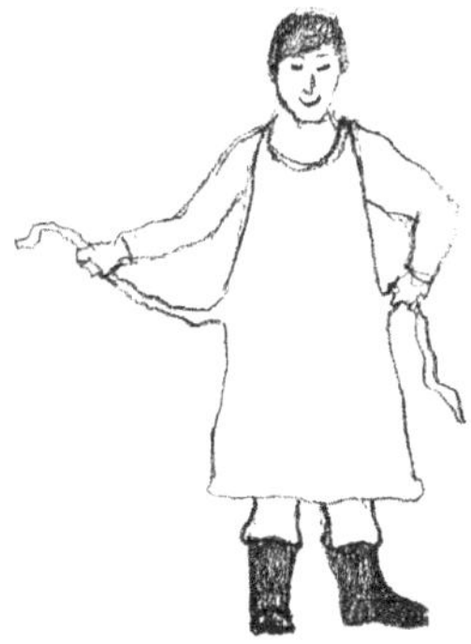

Workers should have clean clothing and equipment.

At the end of the day, all equipment, aprons and boots should be thoroughly scrubbed with soap and hot water and allowed to air dry. Chlorinated bleach (Clorox) added to the last rinse water may be used if hot water is not available.

Access to clean, running water is important. If running water is not available, water should be utilized at the last stage of the slaughter to wash the carcass inside and out.

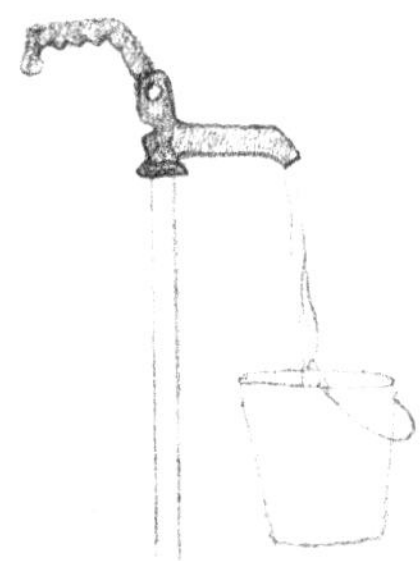

Clean, running water should be used.

The water should be clean water, boiled and cooled if necessary. Water with Clorox bleach can even be used. Water must be sanitary, without germs (microorganisms), that would cause the carcass or meat to spoil quickly.

Cleaning Knives and Equipment

Knives and all equipment used during the day should be cleaned after the day's work with hot, soapy water and a scrub brush. The knife blade and handle should be scrubbed. The point where the blade inserts into the handle should be scrubbed as well as any rivets within the handle of the knife. A hand saw should have the blade removed and all areas of the saw and blade scrubbed.

Any equipment, including tables that come in contact with the animal or carcass, should be thoroughly cleaned at the end of the day's work.

If a wooden handled knife or saw is used, the handle should be sanitized in boiling water, 70° C (160° F) and allowed to air dry. Clorox bleach can help sanitize if there is no boiling water.

A rubber boot that has a gripping sole should be worn, if possible. This will prevent slipping and also protect the feet and legs.

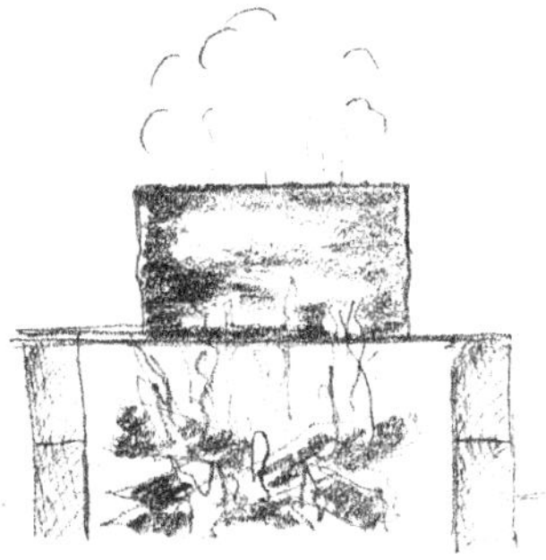

Hot water should be used.

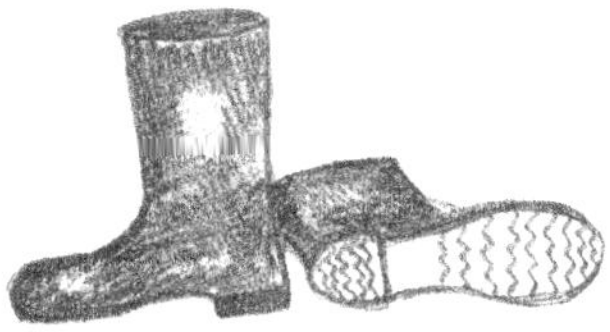

Rubber boots with a gripping sole should be worn.

On the slaughter floor a thick plastic apron will help protect the body as well. Boots and aprons should be clean prior to work and should be cleaned if soiled during the work day.

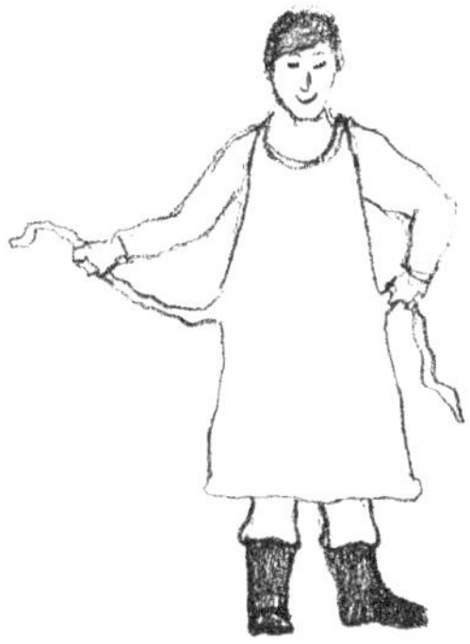

Clean boots and aprons should be worn.

At the end of the day, the boots and aprons should be scrubbed with hot water and soap and allowed to air dry.

Scrub equipment with hot water and soap.

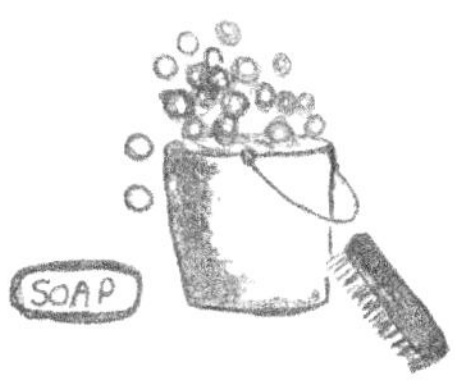

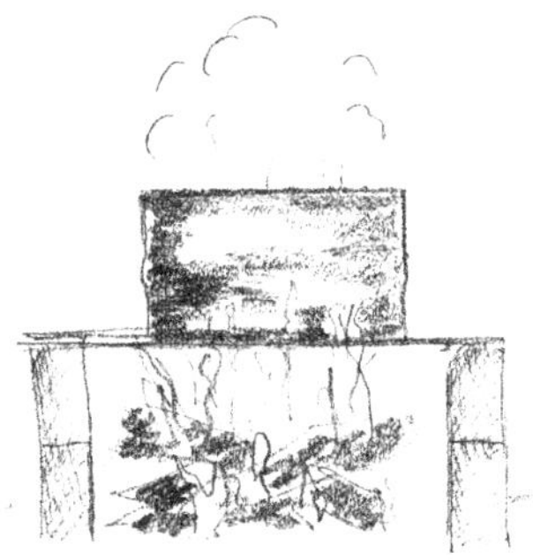

Chapter 2

Knife Safety and Sanitation, Knives and Equipment, Sharpening Knives

Knife Safety and Sanitation

DEUTERONOMY 14:2

For you are a holy people to the Lord your God; and the Lord has chosen you to be a people for His own possession out of all the peoples who are on the face of the earth.

Knives and saw blades are meant to cut through meat and bone. The proper handling of this equipment is critical for the handler's safety.

Knives should be held in a scabbard or pouch that is attached around the handler's waist. The scabbard should have a chain with an open "s" hook for a fastener. This open "s" hook will pull loose if the scabbard is caught and will prevent any injuries.

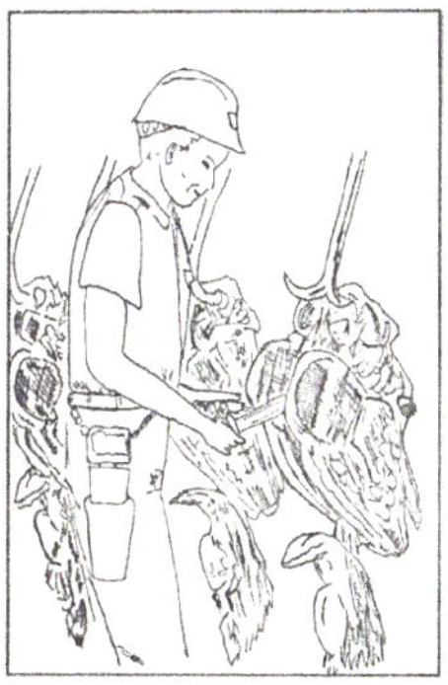

Worker should have a scabbard for knives.
(USDA 1977)

The scabbard and chain should be made out of material that can be sanitized in hot water and air-dried. The scabbard should be large enough to hold all the knives and meat hooks that are used in the process.

A knife should either be in the meat processor's hand or in the scabbard. A processor should not walk with a knife in their hand or lay it down on a table. If the knife is not being used, it should remain clean and in the scabbard.

Hands and knives should be kept clean to prevent the hand from slipping during use. Hands and knives should be rinsed in warm water and cleaned with soap between processing stages.

If a worker is about to drop a knife they should not grab for the knife. The worker should step back from the dropping knife and allow it to drop to the floor. Catching a knife in mid-air could be a potential cut from the blade. Stepping back will prevent the knife from landing on the worker's foot or leg. The knife should be inspected for any knicks, sanitized and re-sharpened if needed.

Knives and Equipment

There are many types of knives that are utilized in slaughtering and processing of livestock. The correct equipment will make the job move quickly and prevent fatigue on part of the user. Knives and saws' edges should be kept sharp and clean.

Different Types of Knives:

Skinning knife 10 cm. to 15 cm. (4 to 6 in.) blade
Breaker (butcher) knife 25 cm. to 30 cm. (10 to 12 in.) blade
Boning knife10 cm. to 15 cm. (4 to 6 in.) blade
(the lengths do not include the handle)
Cleaver

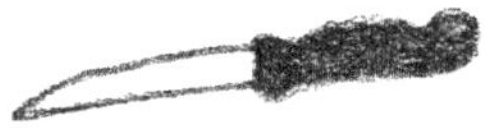

Boning Knife

Saws:

Hand meat saw

Hand meat saw
Electric power meat saw
Electric band saw

Lifting Equipment: Come-along, Block and tackle, Ropes

Spreaders: Gambrel, Singletree, Hog hook

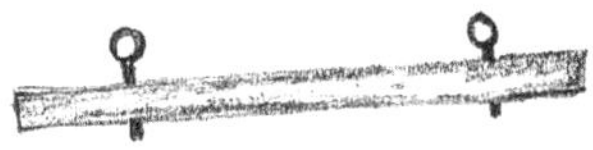

Singletree spreader

Miscellaneous Equipment:

Bell scraper (for hogs)
Sharpening stone (carborundum stone or oil stone)
Steel

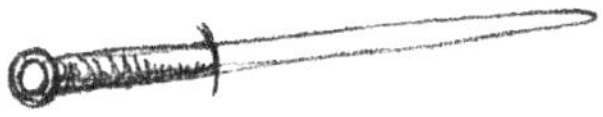

Steel

Table to cut up carcasses (may be hardwood top or hard plastic top)
Stun gun

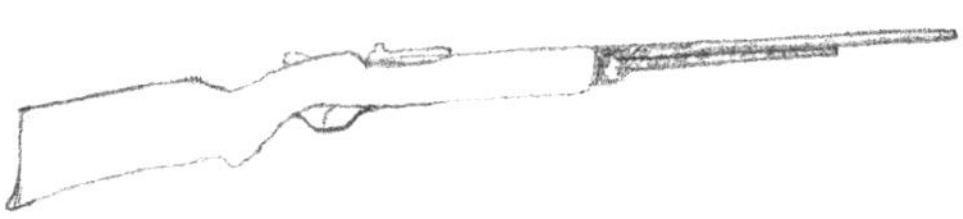

.22 single shot rifle

.22 single shot rifle
Meat Grinder
Sausage Stuffer
55-gallon drum or similar size tank to scald hogs, or preserve meat

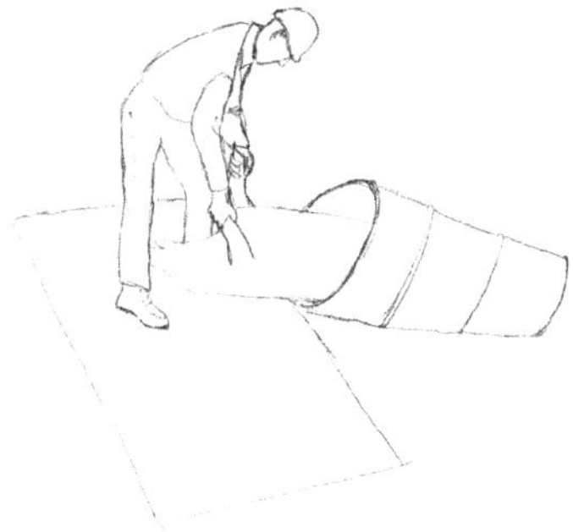

Drum for scalding hogs.

Water hose
Backpack sprayer (for pressure wash)
Bucket

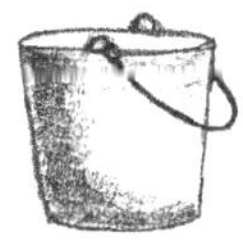

Bucket

Sharpening Knives

Knives must be kept sharp in order to do efficient work and not to tire the worker.

Knives and equipment are available that are designed to prevent fatigue during constant usage. This design is called ergonomic design.

The ideal knife and equipment will be stainless steel blades with plastic handles that are capable of being sanitized. Wooden handles harbor bacteria and will need to be dried thoroughly at the end of each day.

Knives that are purchased from the manufacturer have a factory bevel on the edge of the knife. The bevel is the cutting edge of the knife and must be further sharpened or honed to an "edge" or placed on a grinding stone to form a deeper bevel.

Knife Sharpening

1.Grinding

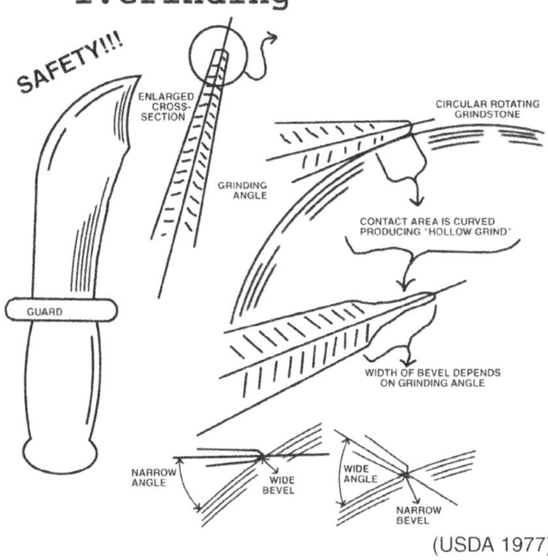

(USDA 1977)

The sharpening can be accomplished by using a whetstone or a carborundum or oil stone. The oil stone may be set in a frame to hold the stone while sharpening. This stone must have a good food grade mineral oil used on it for lubrication. The whetstone or carborundum stone may be lubricated with a soapy water solution. The lubrication helps the knife move smoothly over the stone and to washes away any metal shavings.

Knives are sharpened on a stone that is long enough for the blade to be held at a 20 to 45° angle on each side of the blade. This angle should keep the bevel against the stone. If the knife is at an angle past the bevel, the blade may be scratched and will not be sharp.

Knife Sharpening
2. Handstoning

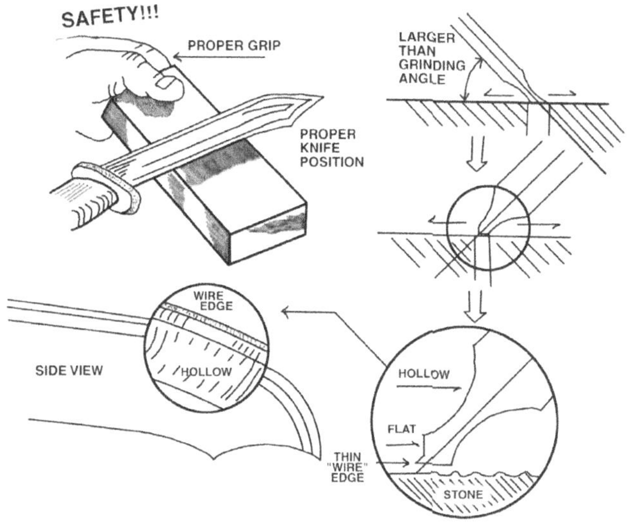

(USDA 1977)

Knife Sharpening
3.Steeling

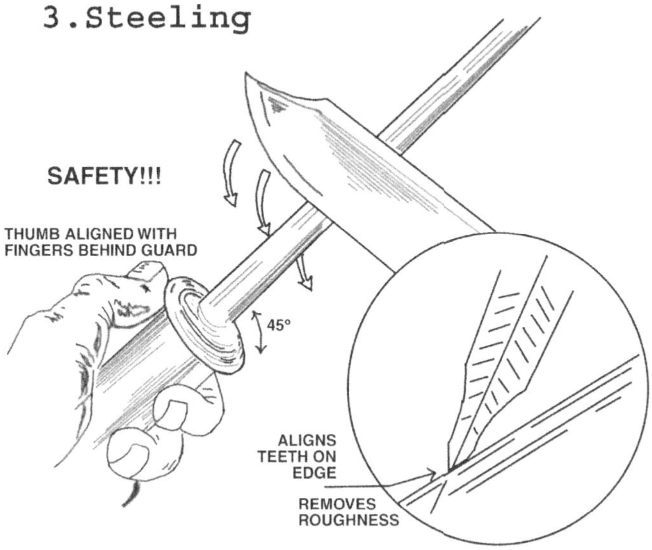

(USDA 1977)

The proper method is to begin at the bottom of the stone with the bottom edge of the knife closest to the handle and move the knife until the tip of the blade is at the bottom of the opposite end of the stone. This will produce an arch across the stone, permitting all portions of the bevel to be smoothed on the stone.

Turn the blade over and repeat. Continue moving the knife across the stone on each side the same number of times; this ensures an even edge.

Sharpening or honing the edge has made the edges of the knife narrow and with fine "teeth", if viewed under a microscope. To finish the edge of the knife, it must be "steeled".

The steel does not sharpen the knife; it just aligns the "teeth" of the knife into one cutting direction. The knife must be held against the steel at the same angle as the bevel and the angle it was sharpened on the stone.

The knife is drawn down the steel from the tip to the handle of the steel. Begin at the tip of the blade and the tip of the steel together and move the knife down the side of the steel. Continue moving the knife down the steel until the base of the knife and steel meet. The far side of the blade is moved to the other side of the steel and the process repeated. This takes practice and should be smooth and lightly moved down the steel.

This is important not only after sharpening the knife, but as the knife is used, it should be steeled often. The steeling will realign the teeth of the edge of the knife after continual cutting of meat.

Section III

Pre-Slaughter

Chapter 3
Humane Treatment of Animals

Humane Treatment of Animals

Psalms 104:10-11

He (God) sends forth springs in the valleys; They flow between the mountains; They give drink to every beast of the field; The wild donkeys quench their thirst.

Animals are a way that we can have milk and meat for our food. Animals should be kept and treated in ways that make them healthy and able to produce more milk and meat.

1. Animals fulfill the protein requirement that is so necessary for the human diet. The animals should be selected for growth and meatiness. Animals should be fed and watered adequately up to slaughter time. Animals should have shelter from the hot sun, rain, snow and cold winters.

2. Animals should be humanely handled and be in good health prior to slaughter. Animals that are moved around quickly and whipped prior to slaughter will have tough meat.

3. Animals should not be beaten, kicked or hit. This will cause stress to the animal and cause bruising. Bruises on a carcass must be trimmed away and will destroy good pieces of meat.

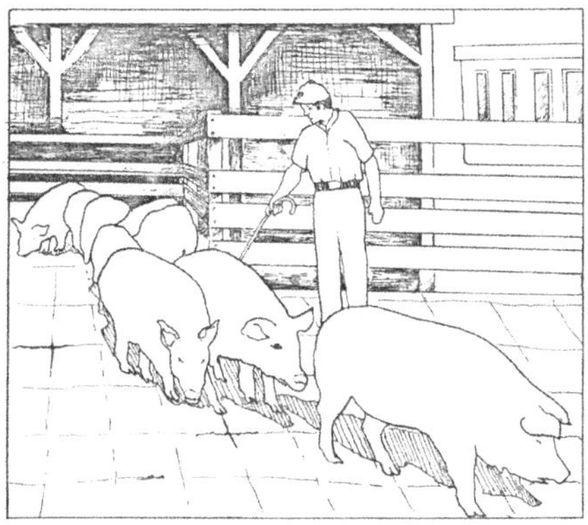

Animals should be quietly moved.
(USDA 1977)

4. Animals should be penned in areas before slaughter where they can move and lie down. Access to water should be available if the animals will be kept penned for several hours before slaughtering.

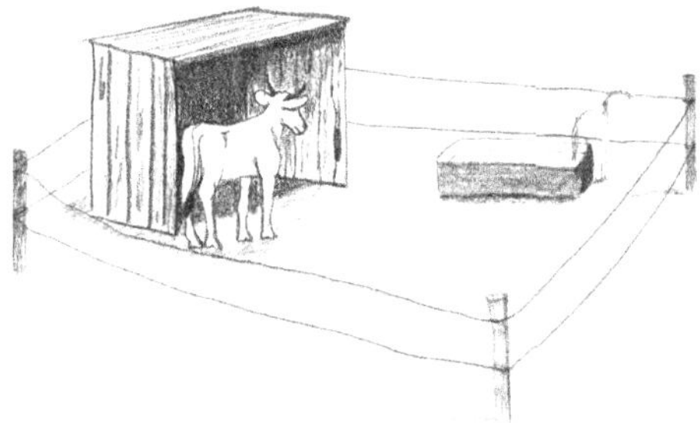

Pen for animal to rest before slaughter.

5. Animals should not be allowed to suffer unnecessarily (not only for humane reasons) but also to prevent injury to themselves and the workers. The method of restraining the animal for stunning and bleeding should be humane. The method of stunning should be quick with the least amount of pain. Stunning prevents unnecessary movement of the animal when bleeding the animal.

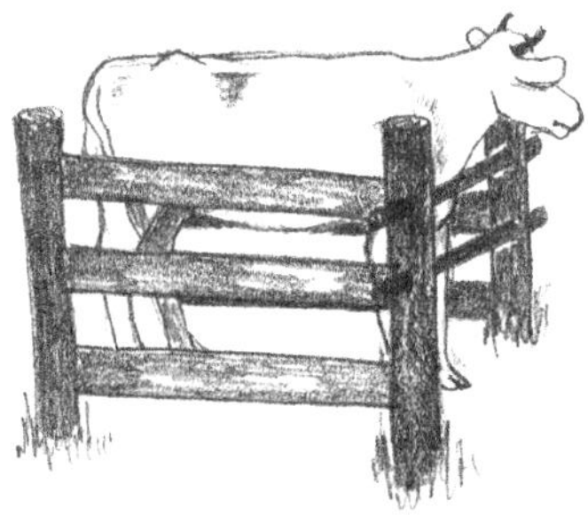

Cattle chute with removable bars in front.

6. In conventional slaughter the animal is stunned and the heart continues to beat. The beating heart will remove blood from the body. If blood is allowed to remain in muscle tissue, the muscle may have a "blood-shot" appearance and will easily spoil.

7. Animals that are to be slaughtered should be kept in a safe enclosure. Free roaming livestock or other animals should not be allowed near the slaughter animals. This will prevent distress and injury to the animals being slaughtered.

Chapter 4

Ante-mortem Inspection of Animals for Slaughter

Ante-mortem Inspection of Animals for Slaughter

Genesis 9:2-3

And the fear of you and the terror of you shall be on every beast of the earth and on every bird of the sky; with everything that creeps on the ground, and all the fish of the sea, into your hand they are given.

Every moving thing that is alive shall be food for you; I (God) give all to you, as I gave the green plant.

1. **Ante-mortem** means before death; examining the animal before slaughter to determine if the animal will be fit for human consumption. Ante-mortem inspection prevents a diseased or dirty animal from contaminating the slaughter floor.

2. If an animal is obviously not in good health, it should be separated from other animals that may come in contact it, until it can be checked.

3. Animals should be rested and easily observed for fitness before slaughter.

4. Animal behavior should be observed including their walk, odors, color of urine and feces, and respiration. Abnormal colors of skin or body parts such as the udder should be observed.

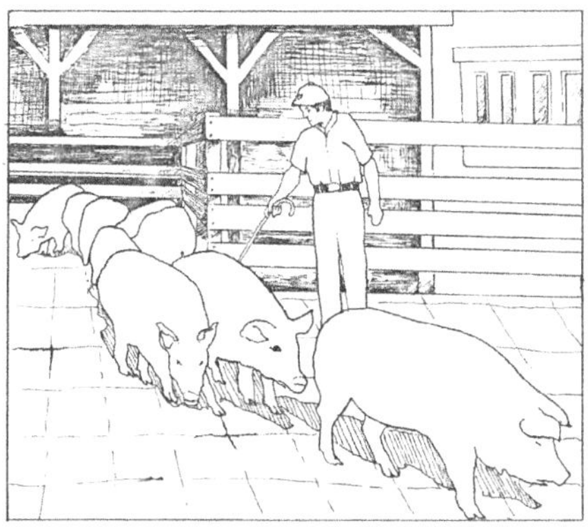

Moving animals to observe for fitness for slaughter.

(USDA 1977)

5. If an injured animal is far away from the slaughter facility, it should be moved by vehicle or trailer, if possible. If the animal cannot be moved by vehicle or trailer, it should be stunned as close as possible to an area where it can be dressed out for human consumption.

6. Animals that are to be slaughtered should be healthy and disease free. A healthy animal will produce more meat for human consumption

7. A dead animal should not be used for human food because the animal may have a disease that the humans may receive from the meat.

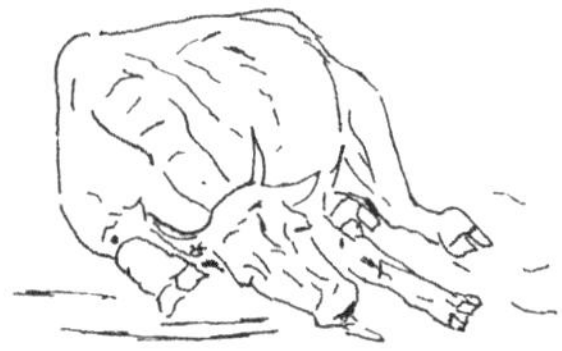

Dead animals should not be used for human food.

(USDA 1977)

8. The animal should be able to freely move and have no visible signs of disease, no blemishes; have no elevated temperature; have no extreme injuries or be dying.

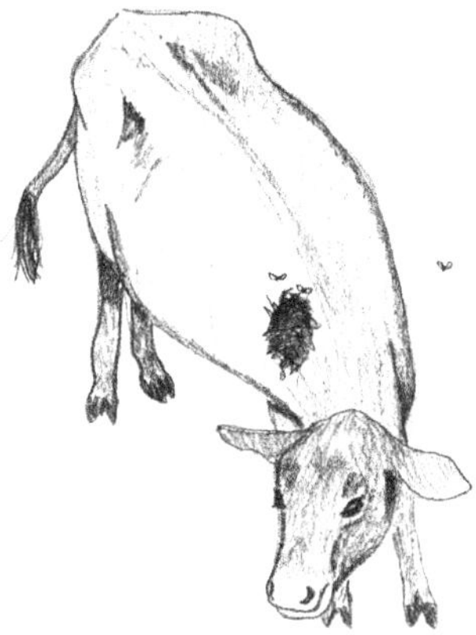

Check for any injuries and free movement.

9. Both sides of the animal should be easily seen while the animal is freely moving. Animals should be moving normally. Animals that are circling or unable to walk or stand should be separated from the healthy animals until it can be checked.

10. The animal should not be unreasonably dirty.

11. The animal should be free from any chemical residues and should be free of antibiotics. This may require a signed affidavit from the owner or animal doctor (veterinarian) concerning these issues.

12. The animal should be moved around slowly not to be stressed or over heated before slaughter.

13. A healthy animal that has muscle on its body will yield a higher percentage of edible meat. Emaciated animals will not produce an adequate meat supply. **These animals should be kept separate and not slaughtered.**

14. Many animals may be slaughtered that have problems such as a prolapsed uterus or slight injuries. Again, an animal with an elevated temperature should not be slaughtered.

15. Animals that have elevated temperatures or diseases should be separated from other animals. A person who can identify diseases should look at the animal and decide what to do with the animal.

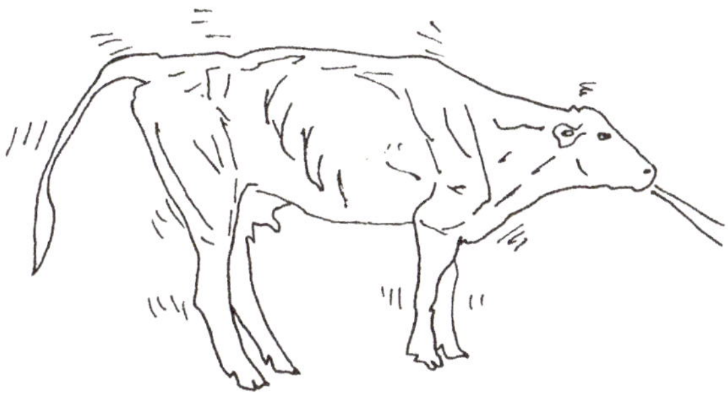

Animals with elevated temperature or diseases should be separated from the other animals.

(USDA 1977)

16. If an animal dies before slaughter, its remains should be immediately removed to an appropriate disposal area and not permitted to stay on the premises.

17. Animals that are about to give birth should not be slaughtered. They should be allowed to give birth and all birth (placental) membranes passed.

19. Animals should be removed from feed 24 hours prior to slaughter, to allow the stomach to empty. The animal should still have fresh water.

Ante-Mortem Rejection of an Animal

1. Animals that are extremely thin (emaciated) should not be slaughtered.
   - **a. The animal may have a disease that could be passed to a human.**
   - **b. There will be little meat will be meat on the animal to eat because of its thin condition.**

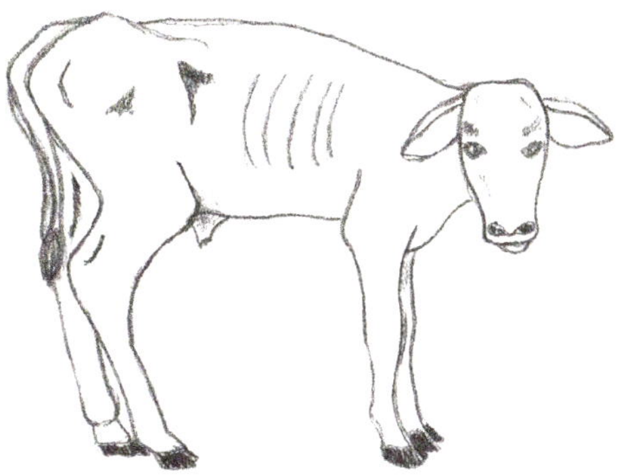

Thin (emaciated) animals should NOT be slaughtered.

2. Animals with a very bloody diarrhea (bloody discharge instead of manure) should be observed for disease. The temperature should be taken.

3. Animals with extreme pneumonia. Labored breathing, weight loss, and inability to move freely are a few signs of pneumonia. Lungs will become affected by pneumonia and should not be kept for human food.

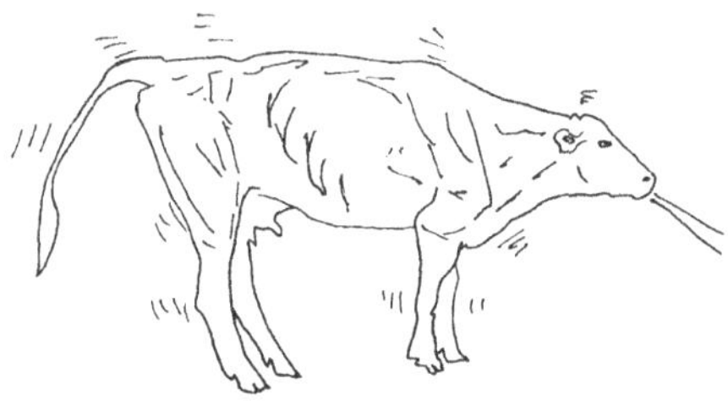

Extreme pneumonia, should not be used for human food.

(USDA 1977)

4. Animals with central nervous system signs, such as wobbliness, unable to stand, swaying of head and body should be held for an animal health official to check these animals. There are many diseases that could cause people to become sick from this type of symptom. This might be an indication to a serious disease.

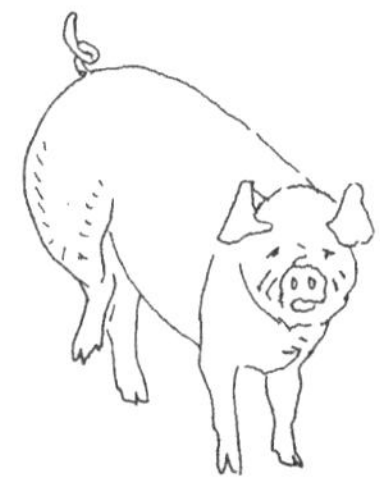

Animals that are unable to stand or sway should be looked at by the health officer before slaughter.

(USDA 1977)

5. Animals with wounds that cover a large area of the body could cause infection throughout the animals' body. This could cause people who eat this infected meat to become sick.

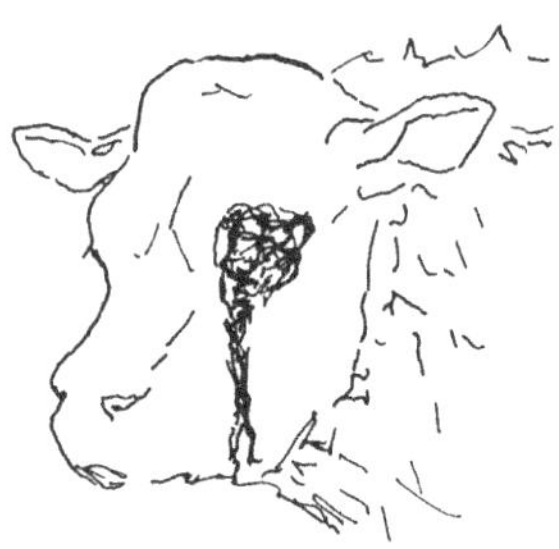

Wounds with infections could go to other parts of the body.

(USDA 1977)

6. Animals with fever, salivation and lameness with vesicles in the mouth and on the feet should be checked by the animal health inspector. This could be signs of Foot and Mouth disease.

7. Normal body temperatures of livestock are found below:

NORMAL TEMPERATURE, PULSE RATE AND BREATHING RATE OF FARM ANIMALS

Animal	*Normal Rectal Temperature*		*Normal Pulse Rate*	*Normal Respiration Rate*
	Average Degrees	*Range Degrees*	*rate/min*	*rate/min*
Cattle	38.5 C (101.5 F)	37.9–39.2 C (100.4–102.8 F)	60–70	10–30
Sheep	39.0 C (102.3 F)	38.2–39.6 C (100.9–103.8 F)	70–80	12–20
Goats	39.8 C (103.8 F)	38.7–40.6 C (101.7–105.3 F)	70–80	12–20
Swine	39.1 C (102.6 F)	38.8–39.7 C 102.0–103.6 F)	60–80	8–13
Horses	38.0 C (100.5 F)	37.1–38.1 C (99.0–100.8 F)	32–44	8–16

From (Tractor Supply 2004).

Healthy Animals	**Unhealthy Animals**
Clear and Bright eyes	Eyes dull, sunken in
Sleek, glossy hair	Rough hair coat
Pink eye membranes	Dark eye membranes
Ruminants chewing cud	Ruminants not chewing cud
Alert and Content	Listless, not active
Normal feces and urine	Watery or bloody feces, discolored urine
Normal Temperature	High body temperature
Normal pulse rate	High or Low pulse rate
Normal Respiration	Abnormal respiration
Meaty Condition	Emaciated

To view and print the illustrations below in color, please visit our website at:
http://www.cvmusa.org/document.doc?id=3089

Illustrations showing various diseases and conditions. (Atkinson et al., 1942).

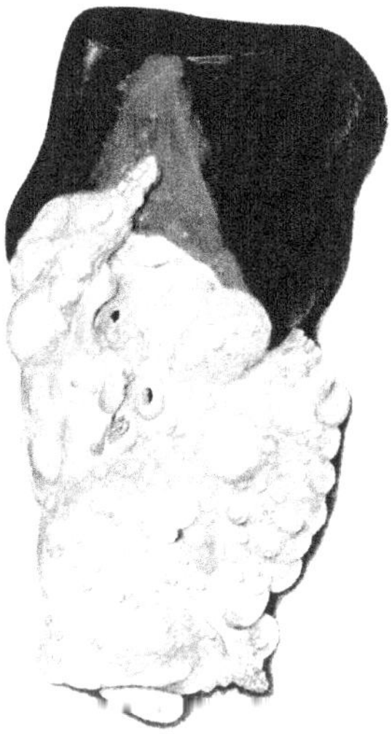

Tuberculosis of the liver

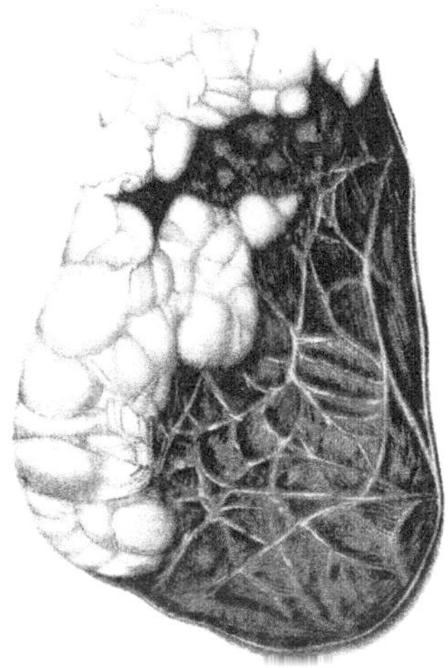

Bronchiopneumonia in the right lung

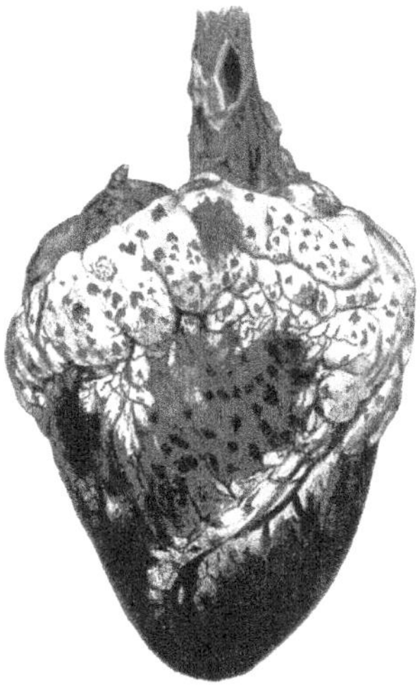

Heart with petechial hemorrhages (very small pinpoint hemorrhages) septicemia (blood stream infection)

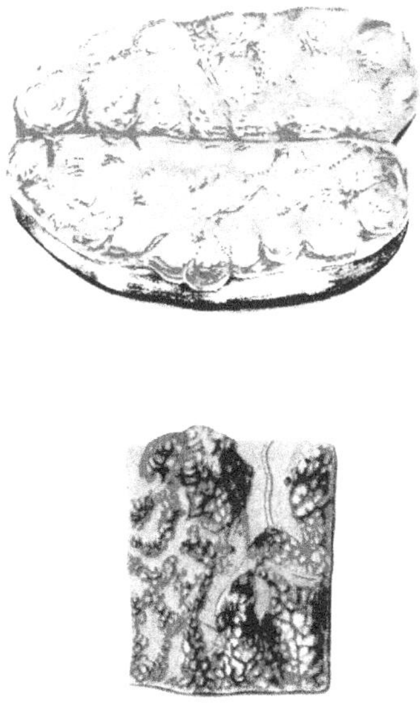

Lymph nodes with tuberculosis

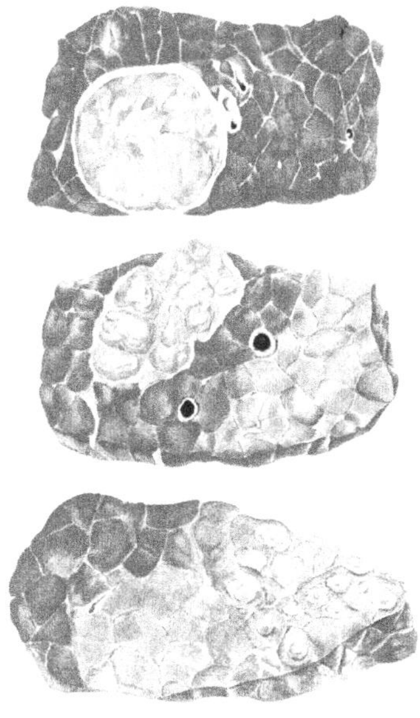

Tuberculosis lesions in the lungs

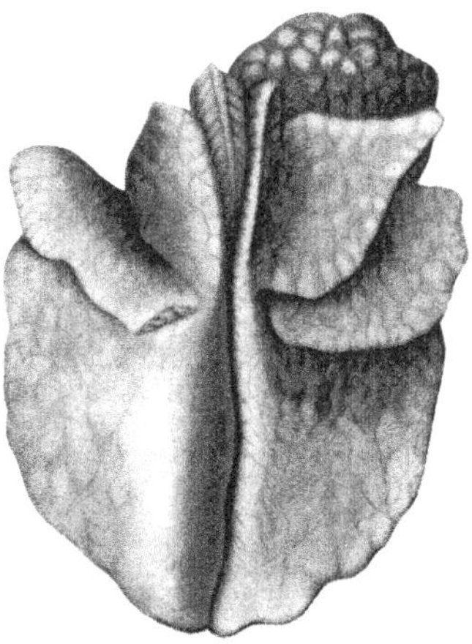

Normal, healthy lungs

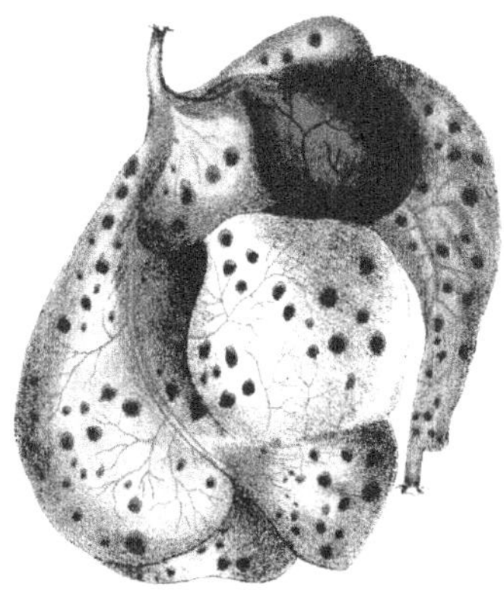

Stomach of a calf with bacterial septicemia

To view and print the illustrations below in color, please visit our website at:
http://www.cvmusa.org/document.doc?id=3090

Photograph slides showing various diseases and conditions. (Courtesy of the USDA).

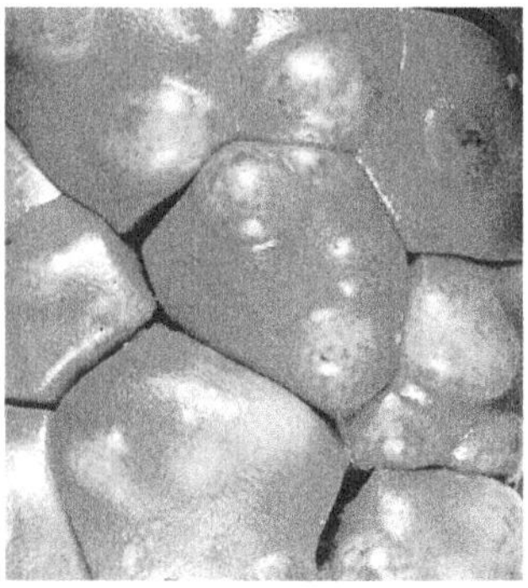

Lymphosarcoma of kidney lymph of 7 year old cow

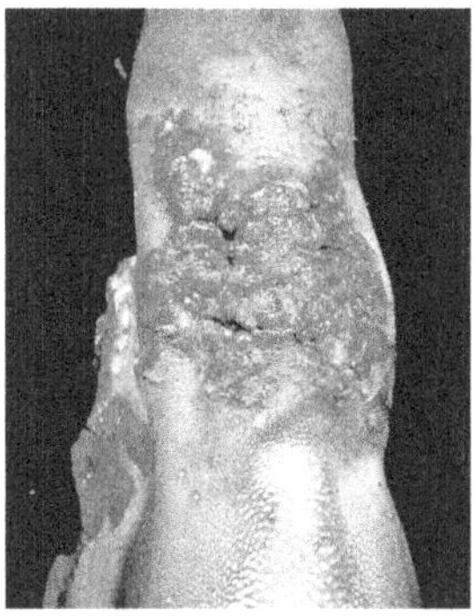

Actinobacillus of tongue of 2 year old steer

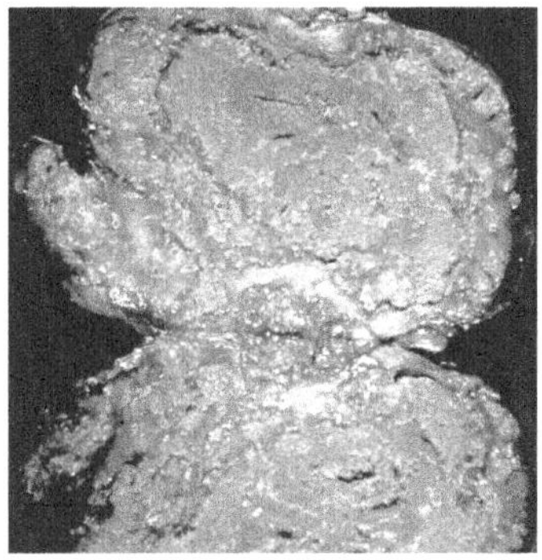

Tuberculosis of cervical node 6 month old gilt

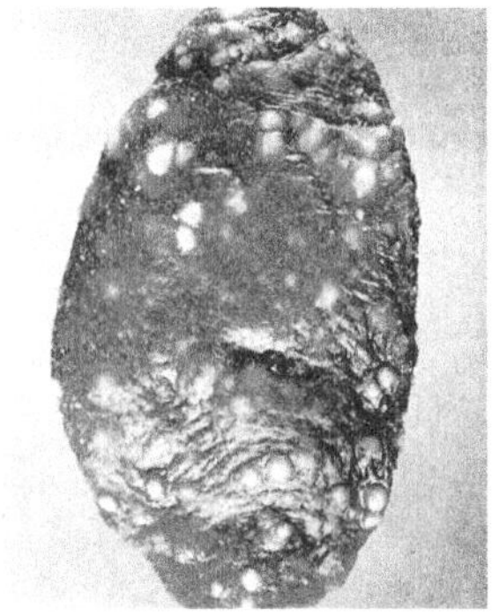

Brucellosis of the spleen of a 4 year old cow

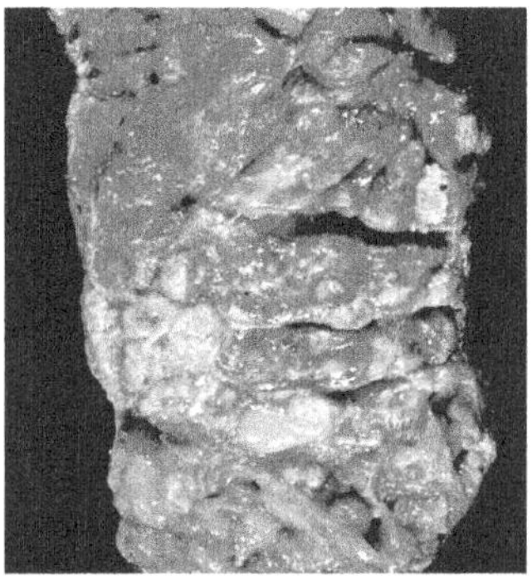

Tuberculosis in lung of 3 year old cow

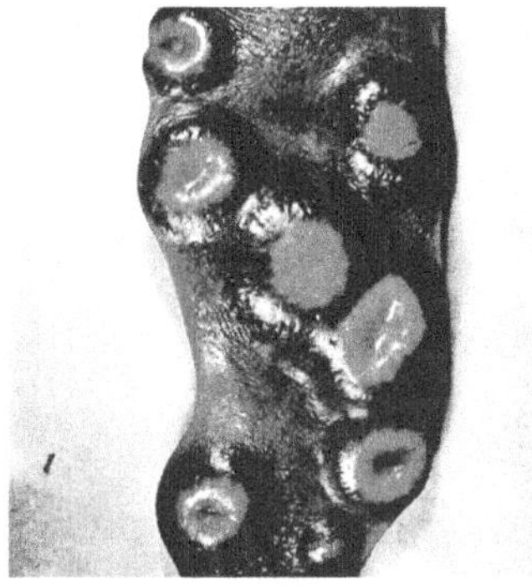

Tuberculosis of the spleen of a 1 year old cow

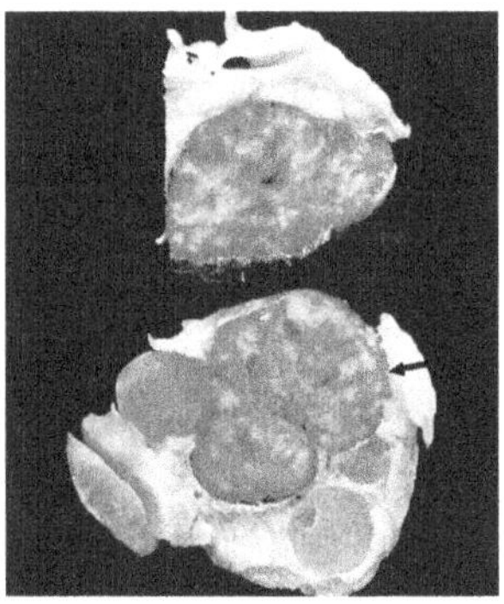

Anthrax of cervical lymph node

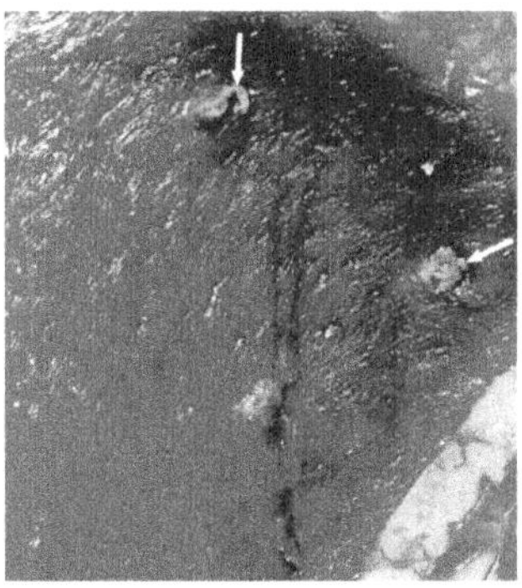

Cysticercosis of heart of a 2 year old steer

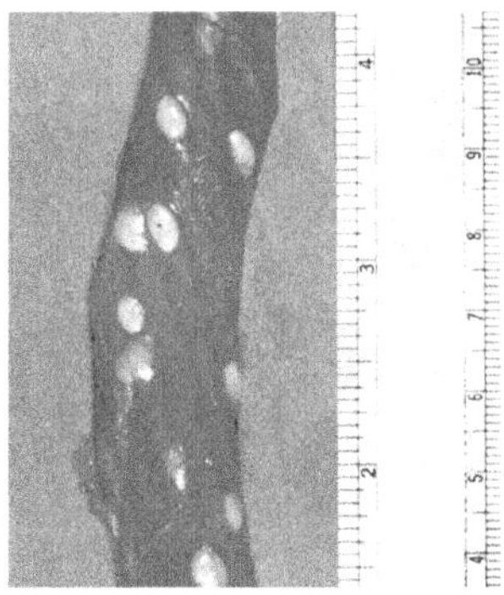

Sarcosporidiosis of the esophagus

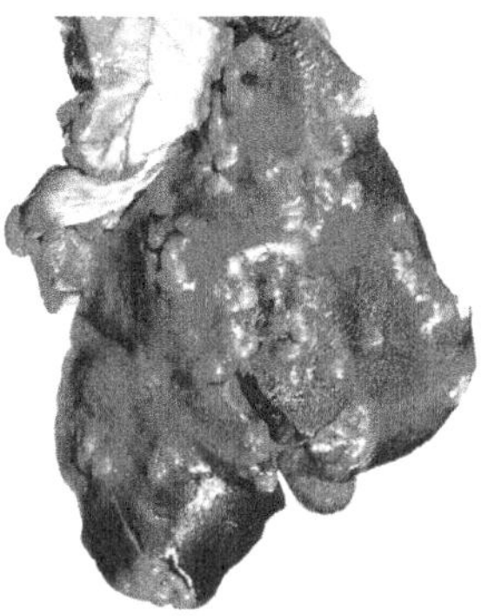

Echinococcus cysts in liver of a sheep

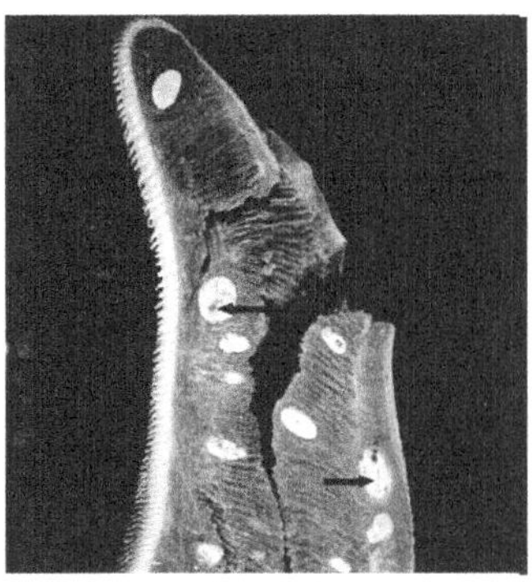

Cysticercosis of the tongue of a steer

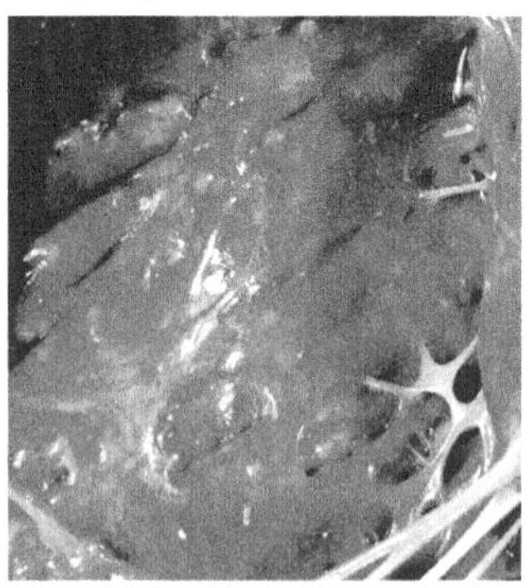

Eosinophilic myositis of the heart

Section IV

After Slaughter

Chapter 5

Post-mortem Inspection of Animal Carcasses

Post-mortem Inspection of Animals

Genesis 1:23-25

And there was evening and there was a morning, a fifth day. Then God said, "Let the earth bring forth living creatures after their kind: cattle and creeping things and beasts of the earth after their kind"; and it was so.

And God made the beasts of the earth after their kind, and the cattle after their kind, and everything that creeps on the ground after its kind; and God saw that it was good.

1. **Post-mortem** is the observations of the carcass after death. This should be done as quickly as possible after dressing the animal, so the meat may be processed and utilized in other ways. All organs and carcass parts should be kept together to observe for any abnormalities or possible diseases.

2. These observations include any visible abnormalities, diseases or other conditions that would make portions or the whole carcass unsuitable for human consumption. This includes looking at individual organs, carcass parts and lymph nodes for abnormalities or diseases that may make the organ unsuitable for human food.

3. Lymph nodes are small organs found throughout the body that filter (catches) germs (bacteria) before it goes to rest of the body. Diseases can be found first in the lymph nodes during post-mortem inspection.

4. The early stages of an affected lymph node may not show lesions that are easily seen. To check the lymph node, make several thin slices across the node and listen for a gritty, sandy, scratchy sound that indicated small calcified scars in the node.

5. Lymph nodes are found on the head, liver, lungs and intestinal tract. Lymph nodes that cannot be sliced should be felt to check for enlargement.

6. The following parts of the animal carcass are checked for diseases and abnormalities that would made the meat not suitable for human food.

Head Inspection:

1. The head's surface and the eyes will be examined. The specific lymph nodes will be cut (incised) to look for lesions, particularly: tuberculosis, cancer, abscesses, actinobacillosis (woody tongue), and actinomycosis (lumpy jaw).

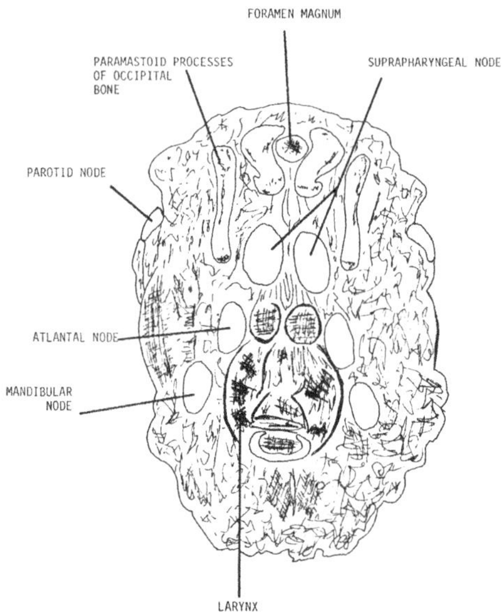

Lymph nodes on a beef head.
(USDA 1977)

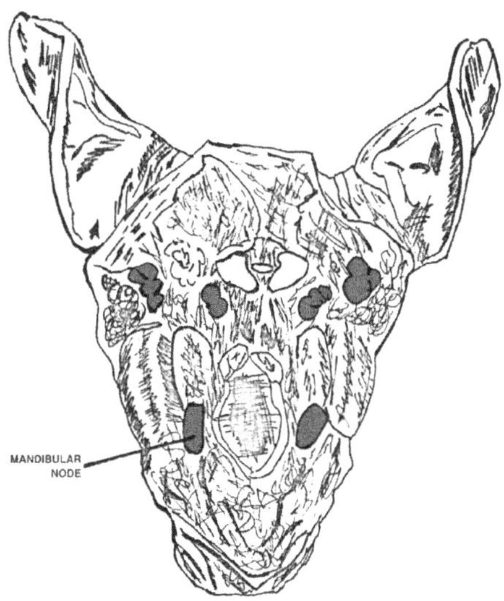

Pork Head with exposed lymph nodes.
(USDA 1977)

Tuberculosis may be a gray, see-through nodule, to a lesion with a yellowish color. The lesions will come together to form a large, yellow calcified lesion. The center of a tuberculous mass may have a cheesy-pus or a cheesy-calcified (bony) look.

Actinobacillosis sites of infection will be on or around the tongue. A lesion will develop with pus. Then as it forms it will become greenish yellow and will attack soft tissue.

Actinomycosis infects the top (maxilla) and bottom (mandible) jaw bones. Lesions have a soft granulomatous tissue and are found on the bony structure of the head.

Cancer (epithelioma) involves the eye, eyelids, and the orbital region. A tumor will be either on the cornea, third eyelid, or the eyelids and will be localized. The tumor may spread to the parotid node, atlantal node, or the parapharyngeal node, lungs and/or liver.

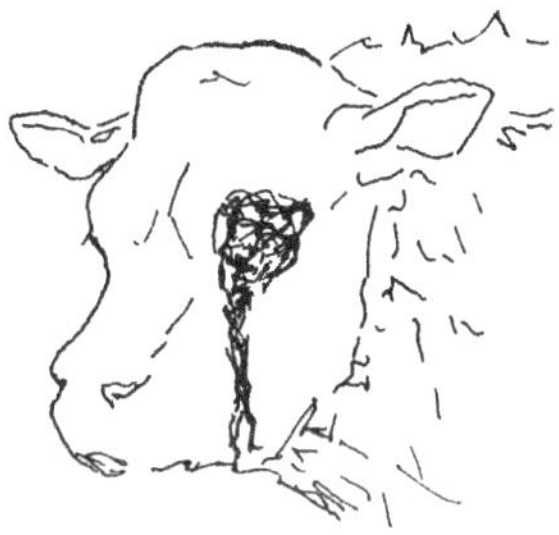

Epithelioma of the eye.
(USDA 1977)

2. Cattle head's cheek muscle (masseter) should be sliced to detect cysticercosis (tapeworm cysts) and other abnormalities. Make additional check for cysticerosis: by examining the esophagus (food tube) after it is removed from the trachea (windpipe); and incising the forearm muscle (*triceps brachii*) 5 cm below the elbow joint.

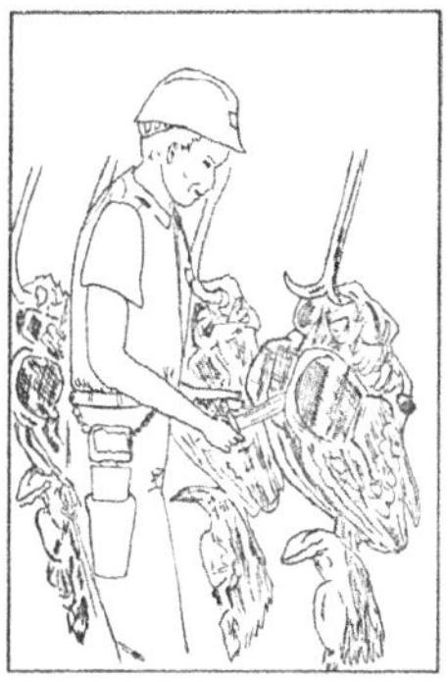

Slicing the cheek (masseter) muscles.
(USDA 1977)

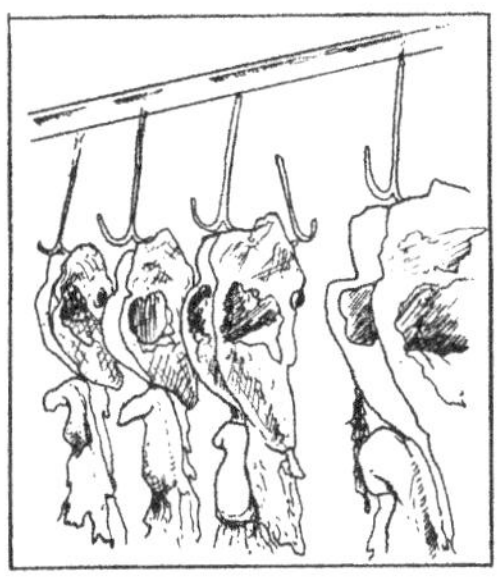

Beef heads with tongues ready for inspection.
(USDA 1977)

Cysticercosis bovis is commonly called beef measles or tapeworm cyst. The cyst is found in the muscles of the jaw, heart, diaphragm and other muscles of the body. It is also found in the intra-muscular connective tissue and is surrounded by a thin capsule. Live cysts are white and filled with a fluid material. A degenerated (dead) cyst had a thickened wall and may be calcified (bony looking).

Eosinophilic myositis may be found in fattened steers or heifers. Lesions may be found in the cheeks, tongue, hearts and diaphragm. The lesions may be spindle shaped and vary in size. They are white, yellow green or gray and may be single or many lesions together.

Xanthosis is a darkening of spots throughout muscle tissue. An excessive amount of a pigment called xanthon causes this condition and also chronic wasting disease.

3. The tongue should be removed from the head and felt along the full length. Abnormalities that may be felt would be actinobacillosis (woody tongue), ulcers and abscesses from hair or thorns.

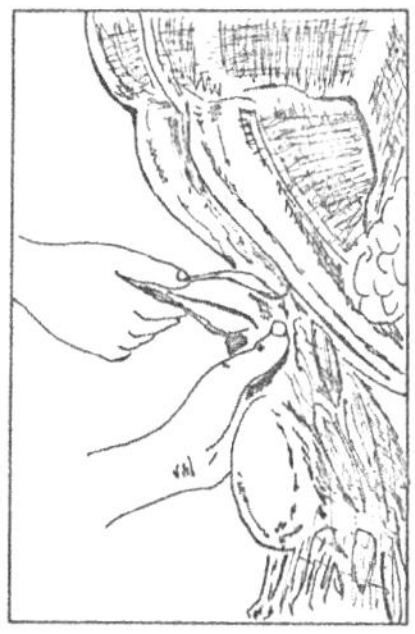

Checking the tongue for abcesses.
(USDA 1977)

Liver Inspection

1. Livers should be observed on both sides and felt (palpated) on both sides to feel for lesions.

2. One or two small lesions may be trimmed and the liver re-evaluated for animal food. If there are too many lesions or abcesses, the liver must be condemned and not used for human food.

3. Hydatids are parasites that form tumors on livers, lungs and other organs. This must be burned so other animals cannot eat the parasite in the liver, lungs or other organs.

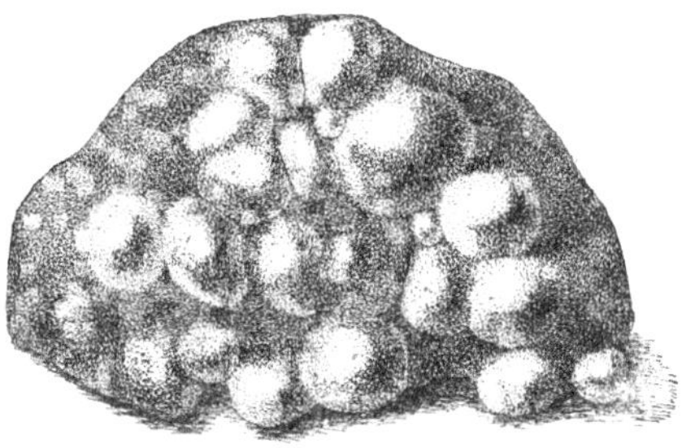

Hydatids' tumors on the liver.
(Atkinson et al. 1942)

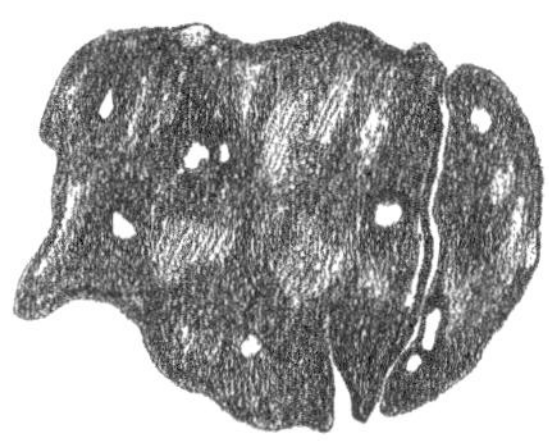

Pork liver with tapeworm cysts.

4. Abcesses of the liver should be evaluated (with the entire carcass) by a trained food inspector. Abcesses could also be from tuberculosis.

5. Cirrhosis is a hard, misshapen liver full of scar tissue. The liver may be enlarged and must not be used for human food.

6. Telangiectasis is a liver condition found frequently in older cows. The lesions on the liver will be bluish black. Livers with slight telangiectasis may be trimmed and used for human food after re-inspection. Livers that are severely affected must be condemned and used only for animal food.

7. Spotted livers in pork may be from ascariasis (roundworm) larva and severely spotted livers must be condemned.

8. The bile duct should be opened both directions to observe for liver flukes. Liver flukes are found in all animals and cause damage to the liver and to the animal. Liver flukes are leaf shaped and range in sizes from 30 mm long to 12 mm wide up to 9 cm long. Livers with flukes are condemned and not used for human food.

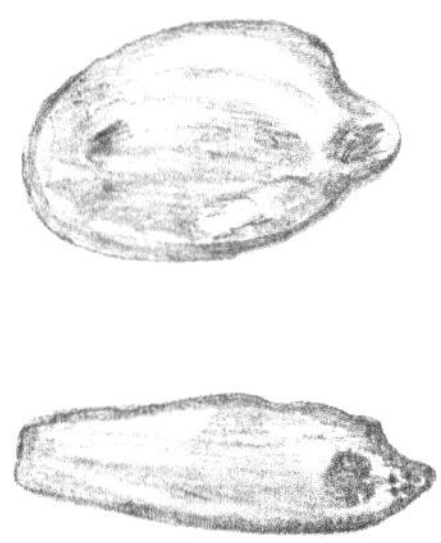

Liver flukes found in the bile duct of the liver.

9. The lymph nodes (one to two portal lymph nodes) may be incised for observation of abnormalities.

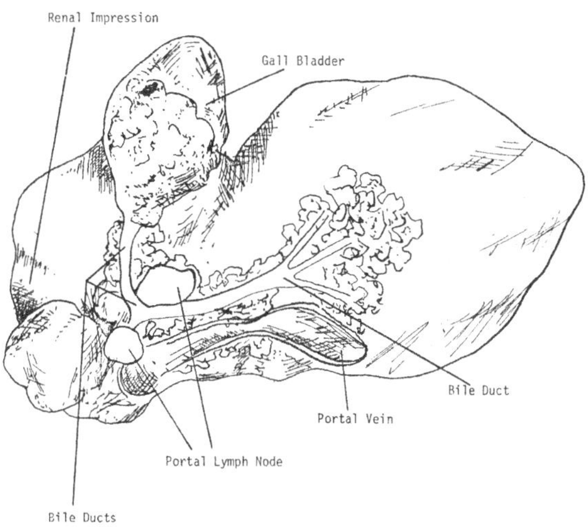

Beef liver with lymph nodes and bile duct.

(USDA 1977)

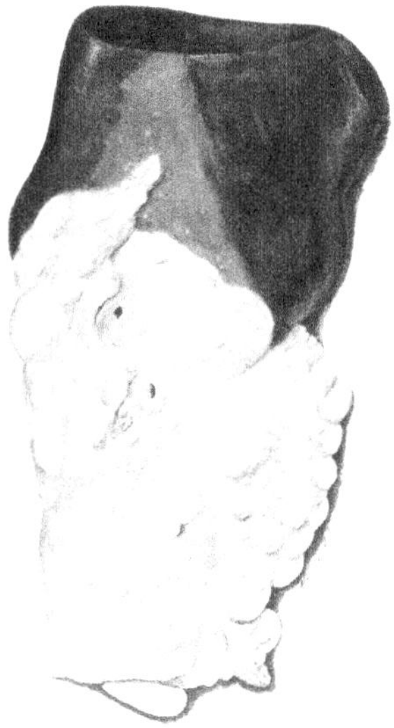

Tuberculosis of the Liver.

(See color insert pages preceding this chapter for color version of this illustration.)

Lung Inspection

1. Lungs should be observed and felt on both sides. The lungs should have no hard areas and should be a bright pink color. The trachea (windpipe) is still attached and can be observed with the lungs.

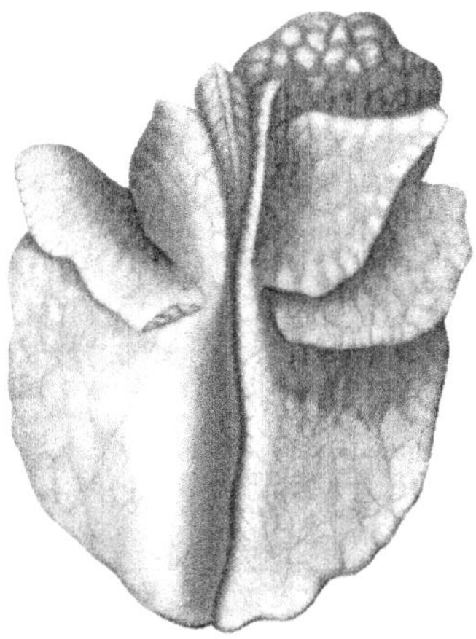

Normal, healthy lungs.

(See color insert pages preceding this chapter for color version of this illustration.)

2. The lymph nodes of the lungs, the mediastinal (posterior, middle, anterior) and bronchial (right and left) should be incised. The lymph nodes often do not show lesions that are easily seen in the early stages of a lesion. Any lesions found within the lungs should be evaluated by the animal health inspector or veterinarian.

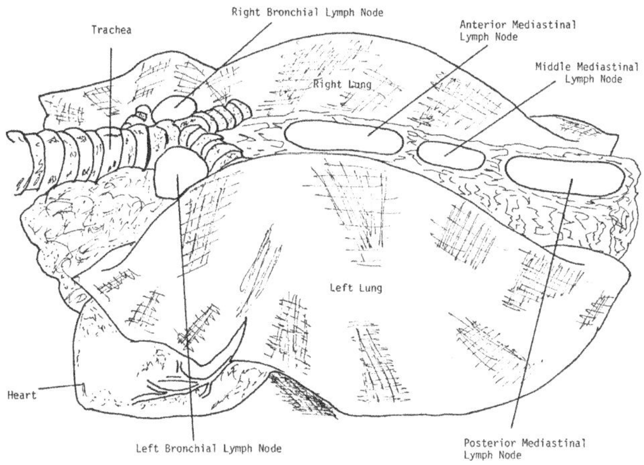

Lymph nodes of the lungs.

(USDA 1977)

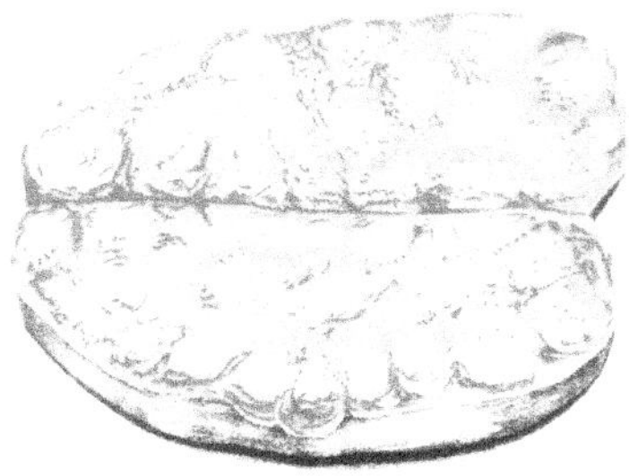

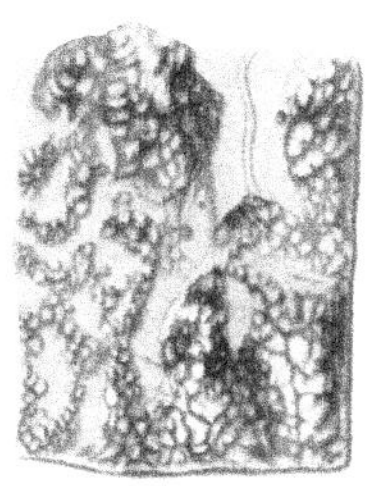

Lymph nodes with tuberculosis.

(See color insert pages preceding this chapter for color version of this illustration.)

3. Lungs that are dark in color and have hard regions should not be used for human food.

4. Pneumonia and tuberculosis are two main diseases that are found in lungs.

5. Tuberculous granuloma found in the lymph nodes will be a well defined capsule with a calcified center in the following colors dependant upon the animal: yellow, white or grey-white. Active lesions of tuberculous will be red around the edge with a mass in the center. An inactive lesion will be encapsulated and calcified.

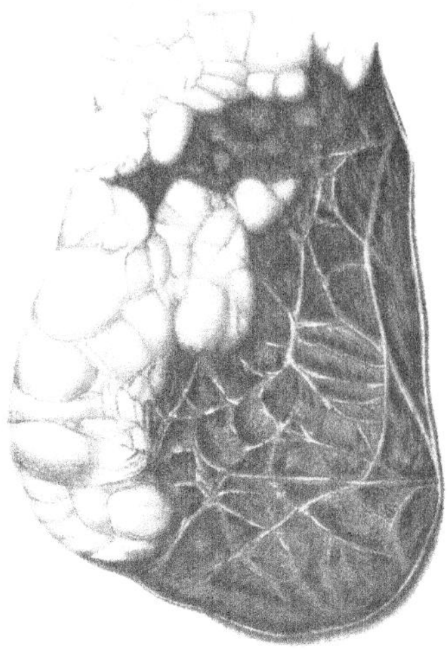

Bronchiopneumonia in the right lung.

(See color insert pages preceding this chapter for color version of this illustration.)

6. Tuberculosis is a deadly disease that can affect humans. Human consumption of lungs should not be encouraged. Tuberculosis will move to other parts of the body from the lungs in animals and in humans.

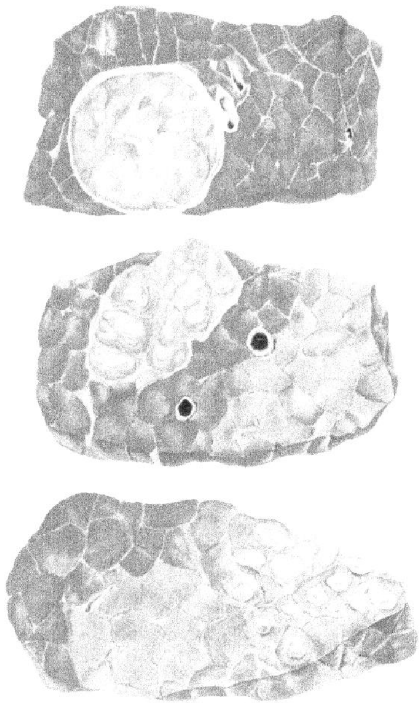

Tuberculosis lesions in the lungs.

(See color insert pages preceding this chapter for color version of this illustration.)

Heart Inspection

1. Cattle species should have the heart opened from the apex to the base through the interventricular septum (the middle of the heart). The heart muscle may then be incised to observe the cut surfaces.

2. Observations of the heart will be for any cysts or lesions as seen in head inspection.
3. Sheep, goats, and swine hearts do not need to be incised and observed.

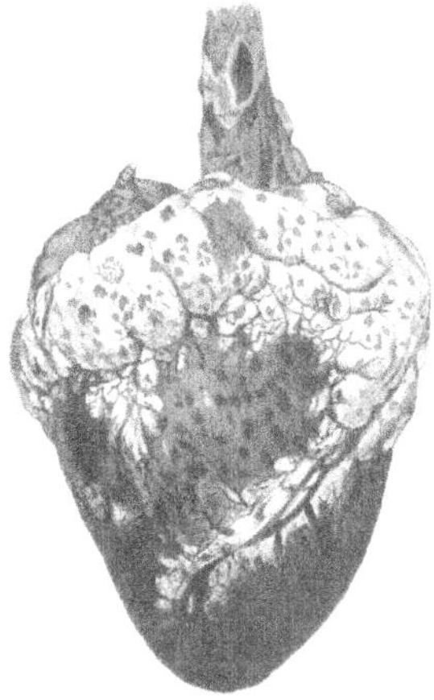

Heart with petechial hemorrhages (very small pinpoint hemorrhages) septicemia (blood stream infection).

(See color insert pages preceding this chapter for color version of this illustration.)

Viscera (Organ) Inspection

1. Udders with milk should be totally removed and not saved for human food.

2. The pizzle (penis) of the male animal should be removed before removal of the viscera to prevent contamination.

3. Observe the rectum (bung) as it is removed. Observe removal of bladder. Observe if any contamination has come from the bung or the bladder. Trim carcass area that has become contaminated.

4. Observe the esophagus being removed. If still attached to the lungs at the windpipe (trachea), the esophagus should be tied with a string and cut above the string to prevent contamination of the carcass, then separated from the trachea.

5. Observe mesenteric lymph nodes (in the fat region of the small intestine), and abdominal viscera. Incise lymph nodes.

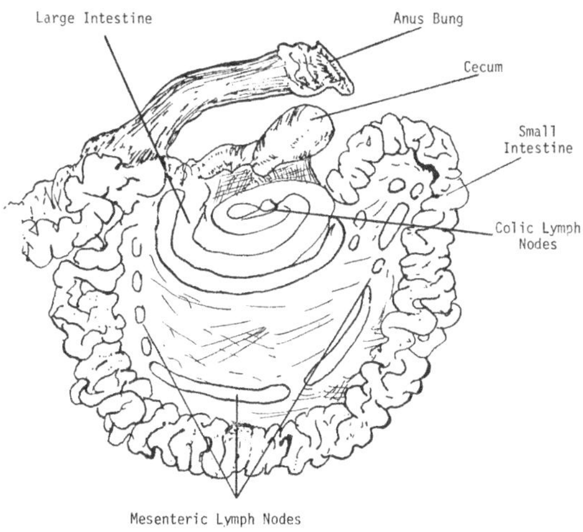

Lymph nodes of the intestines.
(USDA 1977)

6. Observe and feel where the first two stomachs join in a ruminant. Observe and feel the one stomach of a non-ruminant animal.

7. Check for any bacteria infection on the digestive system (acute bacterial septicemia with toxemia). The meat will have a bad taste. The carcass will spoil quickly and be dangerous to humans who eat it.

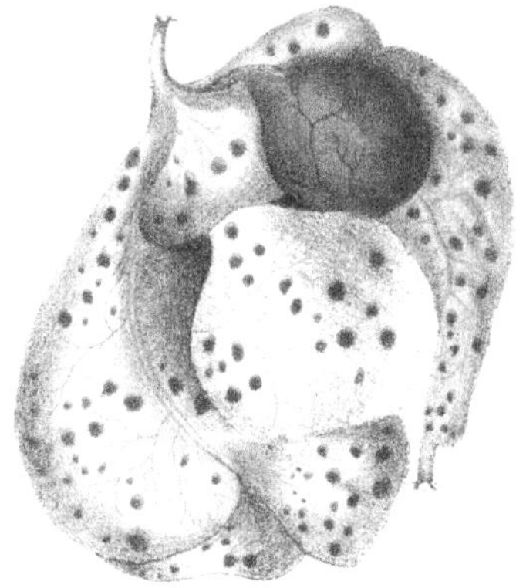

Stomach of a calf with bacterial septicemia.

(See color insert pages preceding this chapter for color version of this illustration.)

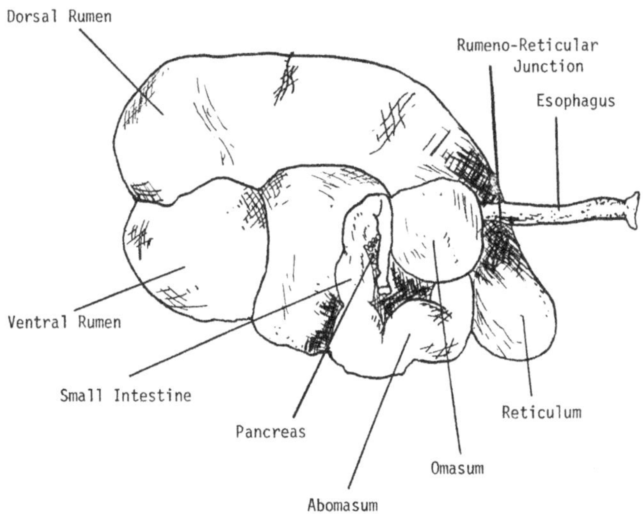

Ruminant stomachs and junctions.
(USDA 1977)

8. Observe the esophagus (food tube) and spleen. Check the esophagus for cysticercosis (tapeworm cyst) and check the spleen for damage or enlargement.

9. In adult female animals, observe the uterus for enlargement.

10. In the intestines, open and check for parasites, such as worms. **Intestines with parasites should not be eaten by humans; the parasites will be eaten and begin to live in the humans. The intestines should be burned or buried. The intestines should not be fed to other animals, because the animal can also get the parasite.**

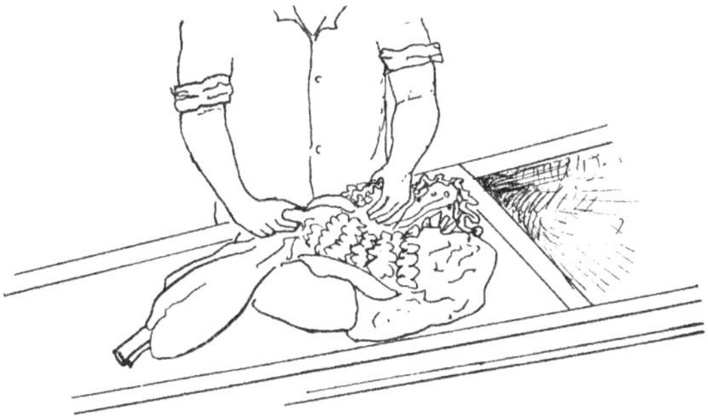

Inspection of internal organs.
(USDA 1977)

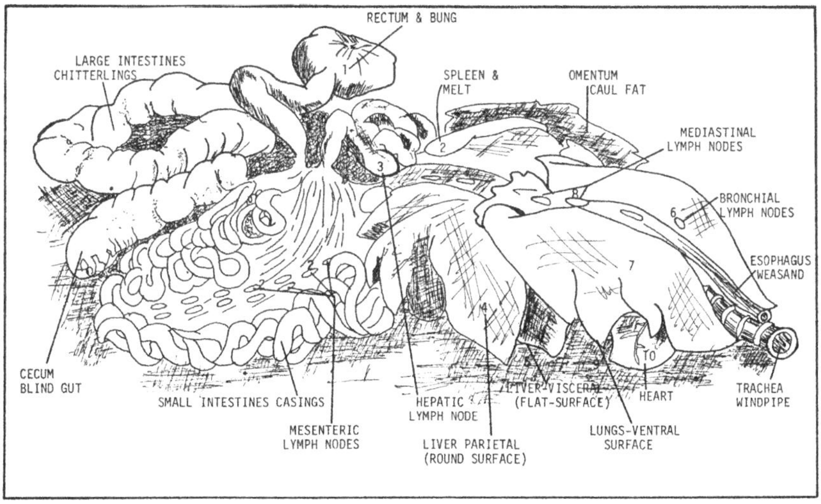

Internal organs of a monogastric (pig).
(USDA 1977)

Kidney Inspection

1. Remove the kidneys from the membrane (nucleus) surrounding them.

2. Observe and palpate (feel) the kidneys. Observe for hemorrhages, degeneration, hardness, or any abnormalities.

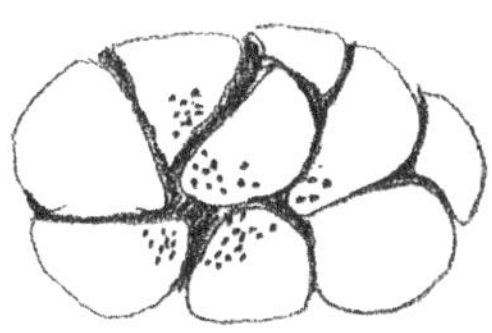

Kidney with petechial hemorrhages.

Carcass Inspection

1. The carcass should be observed for any odors, discoloration, muscle damage, and contamination inside and outside of the carcass.

2. The joints, neck, bones, internal membranes and muscles should be observed for any abnormal color, adhesions (abnormal attachments of organs to the wall of the animal or other

organs), bleeding, bruising, lesions, abscesses or pus, broken ribs, inflammations of the internal membranes (peritonitis and pleuritis) or contamination from hair, ingesta, or grease.

3. Lymph nodes should be observed and felt. The lymph nodes that should be felt include the superficial inguinal (supramammary), and the internal iliac lymph nodes.

4. The diaphragm muscle (separates the thoracic and abdominal cavity), it should be observed and felt.

5. The external carcass surface should be examined for contamination, grub or parasite damage, bruises, cysts and abscesses.

6. The stifle (hock) should be examined for arthritis (swelling of the joint).

7. The spinal column (backbone) should be examined when cut for pus or contamination, spinal tumors, abscesses, necrosis (break down of bone), bone disease, fractures, and tuberculosis.

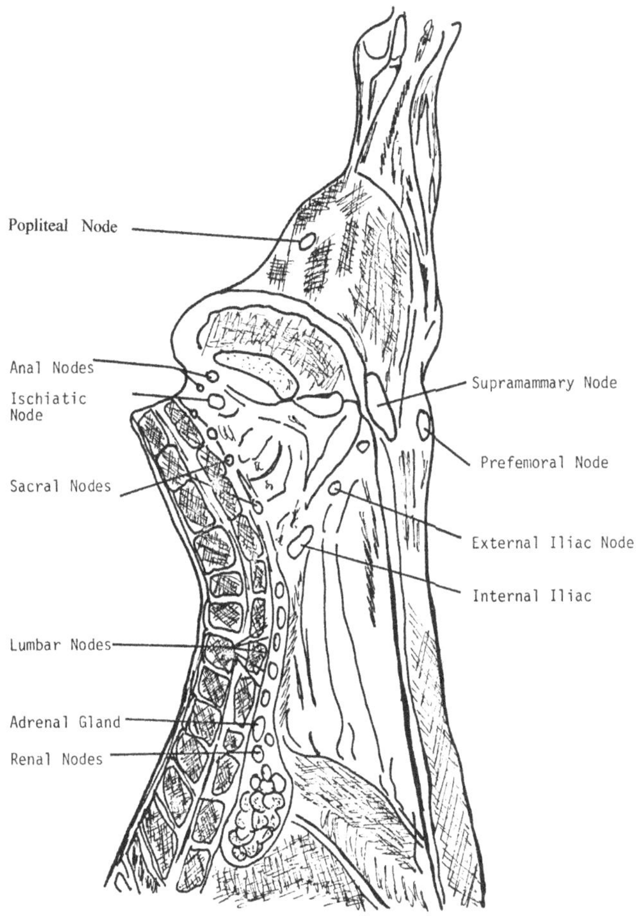

Beef Hindquarter view of lymph nodes and kidney.

(USDA 1977)

Contamination

Contamination may come through milk from the animal's udder, ingesta (stomach and intestinal substances) from the animal, and fecal material. Outside contamination is possible from the food workers handling the meat. Workers should stay clean and be trained in proper ways to slaughter and dress an animal to prevent contamination.

Slight contamination can be trimmed with the knife, and then flushed with water. Do everything you can to get rid of contamination on the carcass.

Contamination can cause organs, sections of the carcass or the entire carcass to be unsuitable for human food. The amount of contamination would indicate the disposal of the organs, sections of the carcass or the entire carcass either to animal food or rendering.

Lesions and Cysts

Lesions may come from any changes in the animal's tissue including meat, organs or any other body part. The lesions may not be seen until the time of slaughter and found in an affected organ.

Cysts are a life stage, or a time in the life of a parasite. Cysts make look like a water bubble or be a white bubble.

Lesions and cysts are important because they can cause diseases in people. Parasitic cysts will mean that parasites need to be controlled in the animals to prevent loss of production, disease and even death in the livestock.

Organs that are affected by lesions or cysts are condemned because of the appearance. Organs with cysts or lesions should not be fed to dogs or other animals to prevent the spread of the parasite or the disease to humans and other animals.

Lesions:

Lesions will appear as a small bump that can be felt or become larger and rounded. The lesion may be hard or soft (full of pus). Pus is made up of fluid and white blood cells that have been at the location because of an infection. This may come from an injury, infection or from a disease.

Lesions may be found on the animal's muscle or meat or on an organ that may be used as food.

Lesions within lymph nodes:

The lymph nodes are located throughout the body and may contain lesions to indicate a disease in the animal. Lymph nodes may be palpated or felt for any swelling or hardness.

Lymph nodes may be thinly sliced to observe for lesions or any differences in the appearance of the node. If there is a suspected lesion, a sample may be removed from the carcass by a qualified person and sent to a laboratory for further study.

Cysts:

Cysts will have the appearance of lesions, cysts may even contain the parasite's larva (worm) within it.

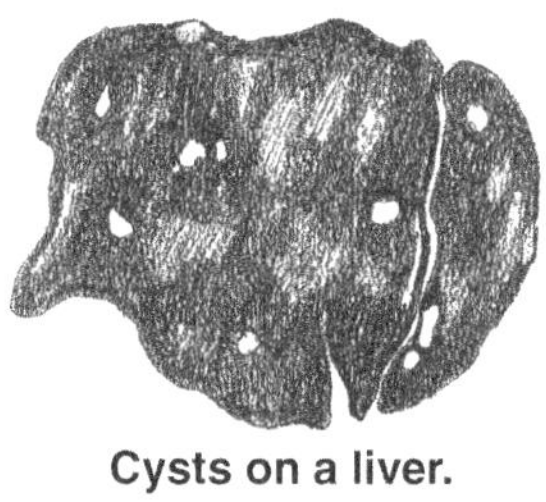

Cysts on a liver.

A carcinoma (cancer) lesion may be located in one area. If found in the lymph nodes, it would indicate that it may be moving to other parts of the body and organs.

A hair sore is a lesion found on the tongue filled with hair from the animal licking itself; lesion must be cut around before passed for food.

A vaccination lesion is a lesion that may be located in one area (localized) where a vaccination was given to the animal. It may be simply cut around and disposed of. If it has gone deep into the muscle, the animal health inspector should examine the area.

Edema is swelling of tissue, this may indicate a health problem.

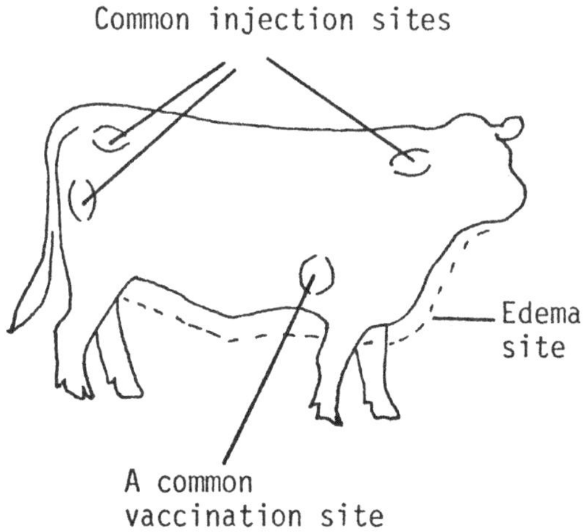

Vaccination and injection sites.

(USDA 1977)

Cysts found on an organ need to be examined by an animal health inspector for identification.

It is difficult to know if a cyst or lesion is from a parasite or a disease. Many diseases such as tuberculosis may be harmful to humans if they eat the affected organ.

To be safe, do not eat or sell organs that contain a cyst or a lesion.

Do not let dogs or other animals eat these organs with cysts or lesions, because it could spread the disease to the dogs or other animals. Then the disease could be spread to humans through dogs or animal feces or through humans eating organs with cysts or lesions.

Diseases and Conditions that Affect Food Safety

From the United States Department of Agriculture, Food Safety Inspection Service.

FSIS (Food Safety Inspection Service) has identified two general post-mortem food-safety categories: (1) Infectious Conditions and (2) Contamination. Food-safety-related infectious conditions and contamination are identified organoleptically, that is, by using the senses, and are presumed to contain infectious agents (bacteria, virus, rickettsia, fungus, protozoa or helminth organisms) that may cause a food to be unsafe for human consumption and that are likely to be transmitted through meat and poultry. Examples of diseases and conditions in each category are listed below.

(1) Infectious Conditions that Affect Food Safety

(i) localized—remove lesion(s) and pass unaffected carcass portions
(ii) generalized—condemn or treat to render non-infective

Examples:

- Abscess: A localized collection of pus.
- *Cysticercus bovis**: The larval form of *Taenia saginata.* Any single cysticercus indicates generalized infection.

- *Cysticercus cellulosae** : The larval form of *Taenia solium.* Any single cysticercus indicates generalized infection.
- *Mycobacterium bovis* (included to support eradication surveillance).
- Pyemia: Septicemia associated with multiple abscesses arising from vascular dissemination of pyogenic organisms.
- Septicemia: Systemic disease associated with the presence and persistence of pathogenic organisms in the bloodstream.
- Toxemia: Systemic disease associated with bacterial products (toxins) in the bloodstream.

* Dependent on other elements in the HACCP plan. On-farm production records demonstrating no cysticercosis in a herd may obviate the need for cysticercosis in the slaughter component of the HACCP Plan.

(2) Contamination—prevent or remove in accordance with establishment of (food safety) HACCP (Hazard Analysis Critical Control Plan) plan

Examples:

- Fecal material
- Milk (livestock)
- Ingesta (livestock)

Part II—Diseases and Conditions with Consumer-Protection Implications Not Related to Food Safety

FSIS has identified four general categories of diseases and conditions that affect consumer protection because they adulterate products but that are not food-safety hazards. The categories and examples of diseases and conditions are listed below.

(1) Animal infectious conditions. Animal infectious conditions contain infectious agents that do not render foods unsafe to humans or are unlikely to be transmitted to humans. *Note: If the conditions are over a large section of the organ or animal, then it could be transmitted to humans and should not be used for human food. Animal health officials should observe these conditions and determine the disposal or the organ, part or carcass.*

(i) localized—remove lesion(s) and pass unaffected carcass portions—only if it is not over a large area of the carcass. Organs with one or more lesions should not be used for human food. It should be rendered for animal food, if lesions can be removed without rupturing the lesion.

(ii) generalized—condemn or treat to render non-infective if there is no evidence of major septicemia.

Examples: Note: these may be passed only if lesions are not spread throughout the carcass and approved by an animal health inspector.

- Airsacculitis
- Arthritis—infectious
- Ascariasis
- Caseous lymphadenitis
- Coccidioidal granuloma
- *Cysticercus ovis*
- *Cysticercus tenuicollis*
- Erysipelas
- Fascioliasis

- Infectious process
- Mastitis
- Metritis
- *Mycobacterium avium*
- Nephritis, pyelitis
- Osteomyelitis
- Pericarditis
- Peritonitis
- Pleuritis
- Pneumonia
- Synovitis

(2) Neoplasia (tumors)

(i) localized—remove localized lesion(s) and pass unaffected carcass portions
(ii) metastatic—condemn

Examples:

- Carcinoma
- Epithelioma
- Lymphoma
- Sarcoma

(3) Pigmentary, metabolic, degenerative conditions

(i) localized—remove localized lesion(s) and pass unaffected carcass portions
(ii) generalized—condemn

Examples:

- Anasarca
- Anemia
- Arthritis - degenerative
- Ascites
- Emaciation
- Eosinophilic myositis
- Icterus
- Melanosis
- Sawdust liver
- Telangiectasia
- Uremia
- Xanthosis

(4) Miscellaneous

(i) localized—remove localized lesion(s) and pass unaffected carcass portions
(ii) generalized—condemn

Examples:

- Bruises
- Cadaver—always considered generalized
- Fetus—always condemned
- Fractures
- Overscald

Section V

Cattle

Chapter 6
Cattle Slaughter

Cattle Slaughter

Psalms 14:4

Where no oxen are, the manger is clean, but much increase comes by the strength of the ox.

Handling of the Animal

1. Stun the animal in the location where the animal will be bled and skinned to avoid moving a heavy carcass a long distance. The cattle may either be in a chute, squeeze chute, or tied for stunning. A chute is ideal and prevents injury to the animal or the worker.

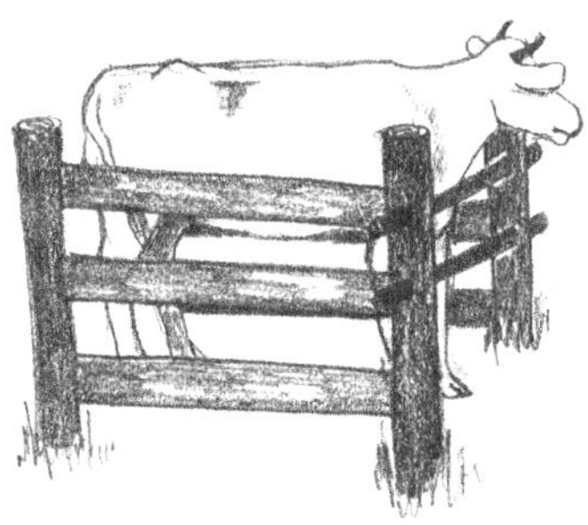

Chute for cattle with removable bars in front.

2. The animal should be kept calm and not excited. A chute should be made that allows the animal to be moved out of the chute after stunning and hung up

3. To tie cattle for stunning, place two ropes around the neck and one rope around one front leg. The two ropes around the neck may be held in two different directions to control the animal. The rope around the front leg may be pulled to move the animal downward, immobilizing the animal (casting the animal).

Stunning

1. Stunning is usually not practiced in many countries or regions. Stunning has many advantages. It keeps the heart beating for the body's blood to be pumped out of all muscles. Stunning also assures that there is no struggling with the animal in the bleeding process.

2. Stunning the animal ideally should be done with a captive bolt stunner. If this is not available, a .22 rifle would be preferred. A sledge or axe may be used only if enough force is exerted to cause the animal to drop. Two imaginary lines should be drawn between the eyes and the horns (or site of horns); where the lines cross is the area to stun the animal.

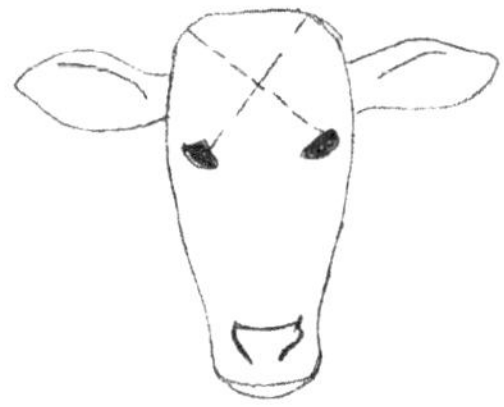

Site for stunning cattle.

Bleeding

1. After the animal is stunned, it should be hoisted with a come-along, a block-and-tackle or a rope with a tractor. A rope may be looped around the hind legs or a chain attached to facilitate lifting the animal from the ground. The animal should be suspended in mid-air by its hind legs. It is easier to come under the animal to bleed the animal, if it is securely hoisted.

The dewlap (loose hide at the throat) should be opened from the sternum region upwards towards the jawbone (mandible) of the animal. Insert the knife straight in and upward to sever the carotid artery.

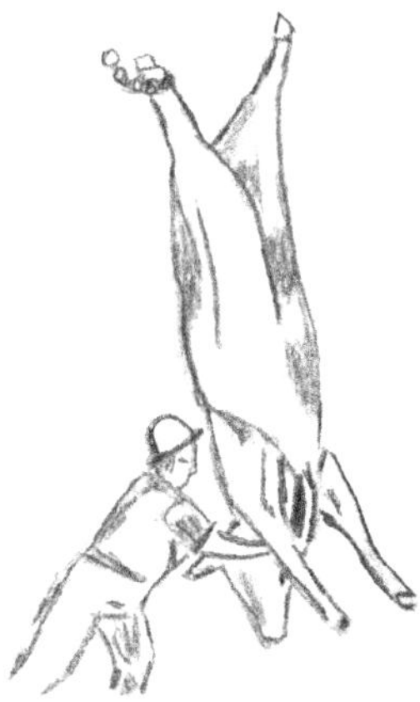

Bleeding cattle while hoisted.

2. If hoisting is not available, the animal may be bled lying on its side. The correct method of bleeding is to open the dewlap, cutting outward to prevent contamination of the neck region with hide and extraneous material.

3. Hoisting the animal allows a fast rushing of the blood out of the body system. If hoisting is not possible, keep the animal on its side with the head slightly tilted to allow the

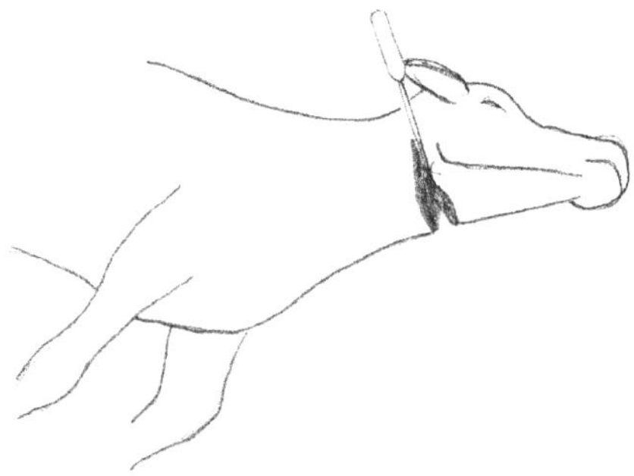

Bleeding cattle lying down.

blood flow to be unhindered. Lifting the tail-end of the animal and pressing on the flanks, may help the blood flow.

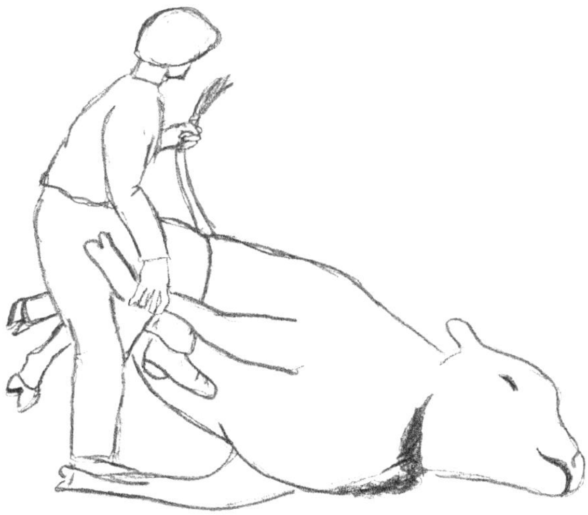

Helping blood flow after sticking.

Head Removal

1. The hide should be skinned from around the head back up behind the neck. The head may be removed at the first joint between the head and the neck (atlas and axis).

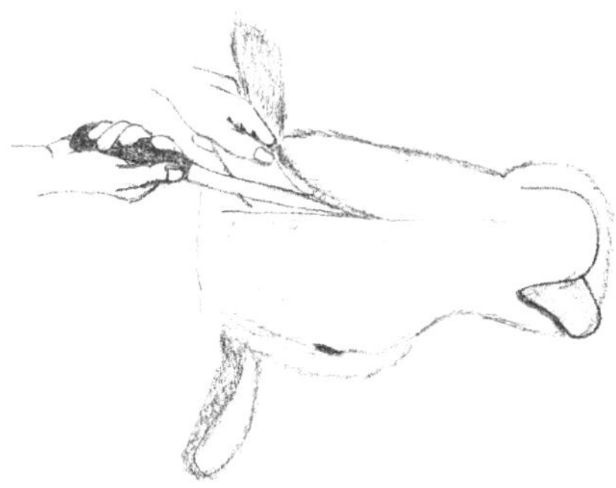

Skinning beef head.

2. Remember this is a joint, the tip of the knife blade can be used to go up and around the atlas on the head to sever the spinal cord.

3. The head may be washed and the tongue "dropped" (removed) from the head. From the back of the head, move the knife blade down and around the mandible (jawbone). The top of the tongue has a thin bone keeping it in its position in the head. This bone may be severed with a sharp knife or hedge-type clippers.

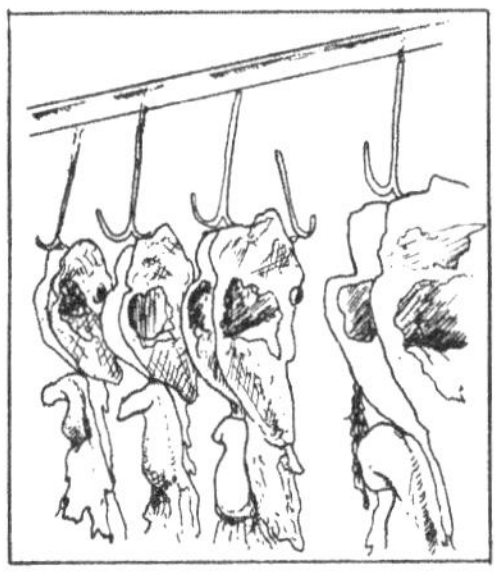

Tongues "dropped" from head to be checked.
(USDA 1977)

4. Wash the tongue thoroughly and feel the tongue for thorn abcesses. If any abcesses are found cut them out. The cheek meat may be removed, also the meat over the top of the head, and used for sausage or ground.

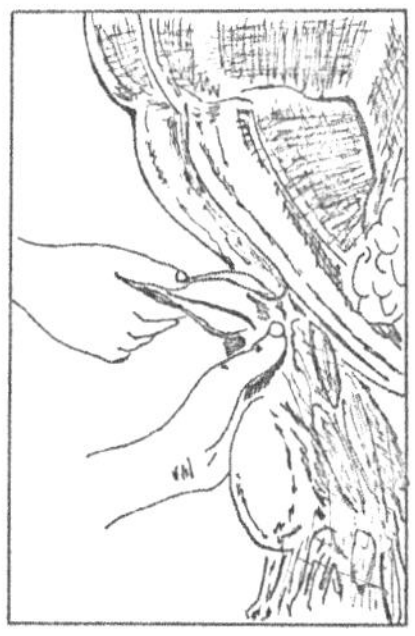

Feeling tongue for abcesses.
(USDA 1977)

Skinning

Bed or Cradle Method

1. After bleeding, the animal should be removed from the ground to the bed or cradle for skinning. If no bed or cradle is available, roll the animal on its back and prop each side with a large brick or weight to prevent it from rolling.

2. Even propping the animal on each side with a large stick stuck in the ground will help the operation. Double loop and tie securely a rope around the hind legs. If a chain is used, make sure it does not slip and is secured below the hock. Lower the animal onto the bed to begin skinning.

3. The hind and fore legs should be removed first. The hide should be skinned free from the bone from below the dewclaws down towards the hock. The knife should be brought outward from the hide. Care should be taken that the knife and hands are clean and contamination from the hide does not get on the carcass.

4. The hide on the hind-legs is opened down the back of the legs down to the cod (testical sac) or udder.

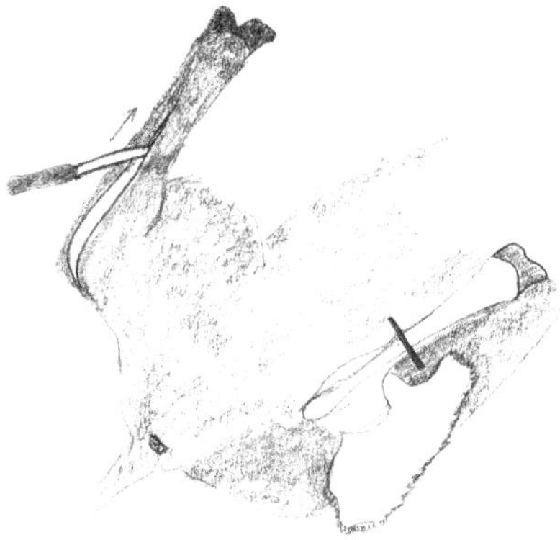

Skinning Hind Hocks.

5. The hide on the front-legs is opened down to a point on the brisket.

6. When the hock is reached, it may be removed at the joint with a knife. If the joint cannot be separated with a knife, a saw may be used to saw through the bone.

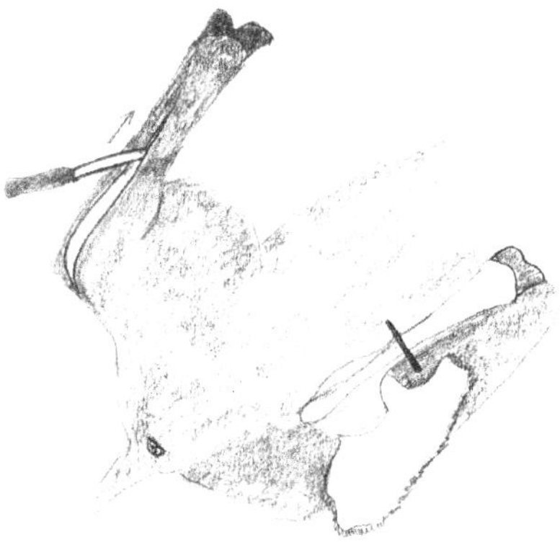

Hock removal.

7. Make sure that the hind-legs are not cut too close to the hock or the tendon, so they will hold the carcass on the gambrel. Hook the hocks through the singletree gambrel and attach to the pulley or rope.

8. After the front and hind legs are removed the hide may be opened. Open the hide from the sternum (brisket area) up the mid-line of the carcass to the rectum.

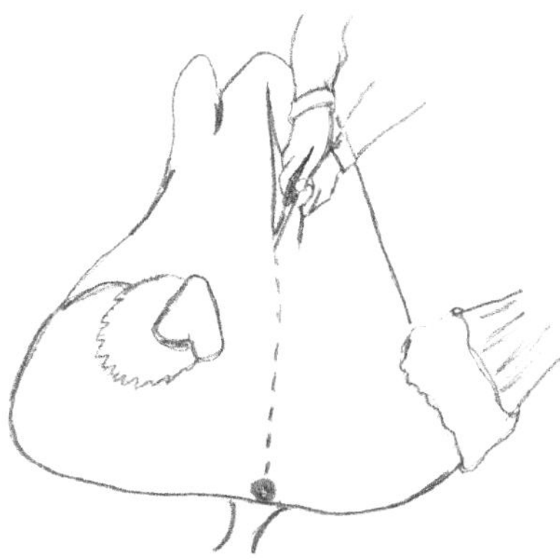

Opening the hide down the middle.

9. Keep the knife blade pointing out and keep the knife clean. Using the free hand hold and lift the hide and pull it away from the carcass as you skin close to the hide.

10. Avoid sticking the point of the knife into the meat; use the entire blade in a sweeping motion.

11. Leave as much fat on the carcass as possible. Be careful around the flank and the round area. Keep your hands and the knife as clean as possible to prevent contamination of the carcass from the hide. Remove the hide off the fore legs and the hind legs and over the brisket. Continue to skin down the side as far as you can go.

12. Before the carcass is hoisted, the trachea (windpipe) and esophagus (food tube) should be separated with a weasand rod. If this is not possible, hold one end of the esophagus and move your hand up the esophagus to separate the connective tissue.

The esophagus (food tube) should be tied with a string, so that the stomach contents will not run out.

13. Begin to hoist the carcass making sure the gambrels are tightly in the hocks. Hoist the carcass far enough to raise the hindquarter then stop to continue skinning the hindquarter, down around the rump and the hip. Exercise care not to gouge into the meat and continue keeping the carcass clean.

14. Before you lift the carcass any further tie off the bung (rectum and urogenital opening). Grasp the bung and carefully move your knife around it to loosen it from the surrounding tissue. Tie the bung tightly with a string and push the bung down inside the carcass. If there is any manure leakage, cut the manure off the carcass and recheck the string.

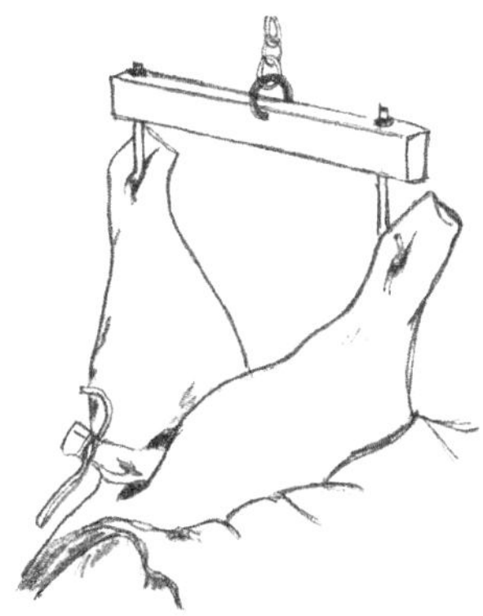

Bung tied and loosened after hoisting and skinning.

15. Now is also a good time to remove the tail. Making sure there is no manure or mud on the tail, open the hide on the inside of the tail from the rectum to the tip of the tail.

16. The hide may be pulled off the tail or skinned off. It may be easier to skin the tail, pulling on the hide could possible cause the carcass to fall off the gambrel. After the hide is removed from the tail, the tail may be cut off at a joint close to the carcass.

17. Wash the tail thoroughly.

18. Lift the carcass and open the abdominal cavity in front of the pelvis. Do not go in far enough to rupture the intestines. Lift the carcass higher and hold the knife with the blade sticking out of the opening to the abdomen. Keep the heel of the knife against the inside of the midline of the abdomen. Continue to move the knife down the midline from the pelvic area to the rear part of the breastbone.

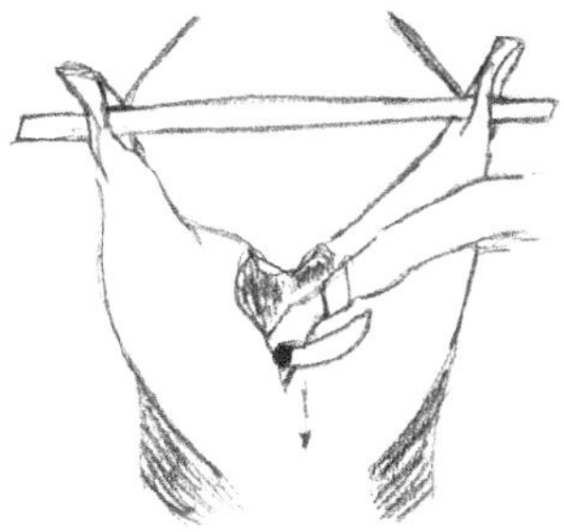

Opening abdominal cavity knife pointing outward and moving downward.

19. Continue to move the carcass up off the ground. Remove the hide down to the forequarter to protect the carcass from getting dirty. Saw through the pelvic bone to open up the pelvic cavity.

Evisceration (Removal of organs)

1. Go back up to the pelvic area and grasping the bung pull it straight out of the carcass.
2. When coming to the bladder, remove it to prevent spillage.

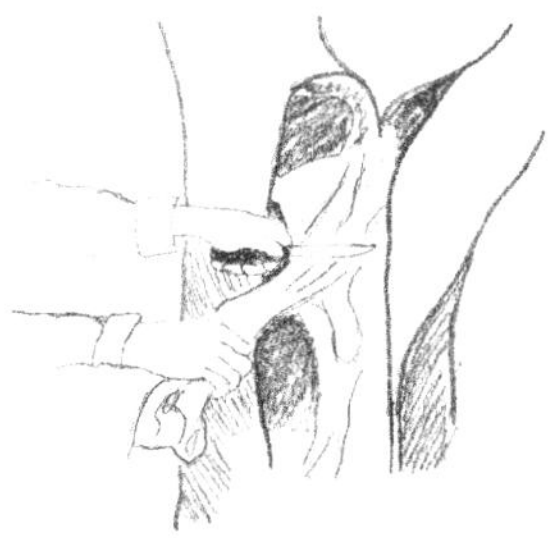

Pulling bung out and removing bladder.

3. Continue cutting the tissue behind the intestines and pull the intestines out. When reaching the rumen (large stomach), the intestines should roll out of the carcass.

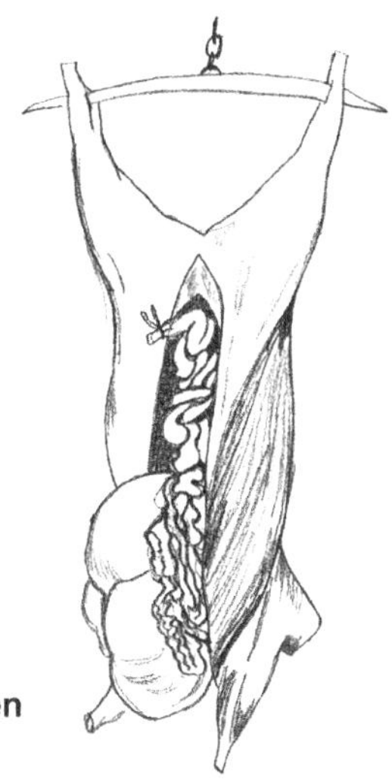

Intestines fall out when rumen is pulled out.

4. Leave the kidneys in the carcass. The liver should be removed from the organs (viscera). Remove the liver by pulling it away from the body's attachments. Separate the gall bladder from the liver and wash the liver.

5. Remove the rumen and free the esophagus as it comes up through the diaphragm (muscle that separates the top thoracic cavity from the bottom abdominal cavity).

6. Open the breastbone (sternum) and cut around the diaphragm close to the body and remove the lungs and heart (pluck) with the trachea. The trachea and the esophagus may not have pulled out entirely from the region of the neck where the animal was bled.

7. Remove the heart from the lungs, cut open the heart to remove blood clots, examine for disease, and rinse well.

8. Check the inside of the carcass for any remaining ingesta (stomach, gut contents) or manure. Trim the contamination with a knife before washing. The kidneys can be removed from the fat and the membrane surrounding them. The kidneys can be examined.

Splitting the Carcass

1. Open up the pelvic bone with a saw, from the inside of the carcass. This will make it easier to split (saw into two halves) the beef carcass.

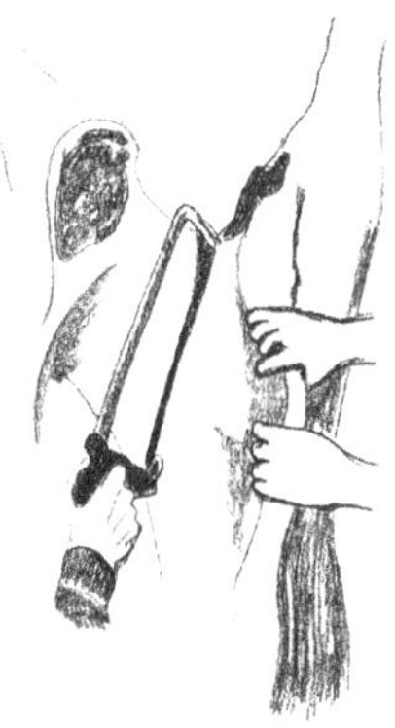

Sawing pelvic bone from inside the carcass.

2. Split the carcass by sawing down the length of the backbone. Follow the backbone down, preventing the saw from cutting into the ribeye muscle.

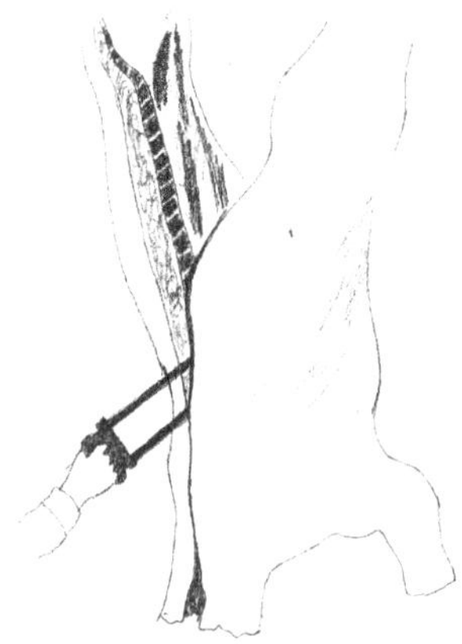

Splitting the carcass down the backbone.

Washing and Cooling the Carcass

1. The carcass should be washed inside and out making sure that the carcass has no contamination of hair and ingesta. Hang the carcass where it can be kept cool until time to cut the carcass.

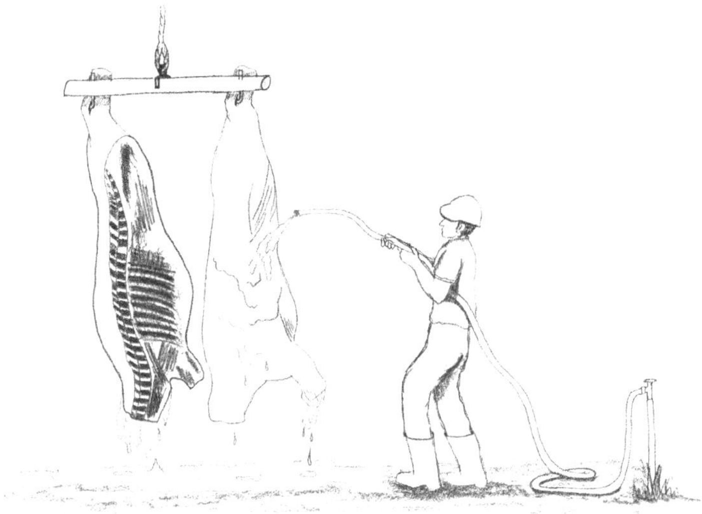

Washing the carcass inside and out.

2. If the carcass will be utilized as a ground product or as a sausage, the carcass may be boned out "hot" or unchilled. This saves on the cost of refrigeration and the whole process of slaughter and processing may be done at one time. The process for hot boning is at the beginning of the section on beef processing.

By-products and hides

1. By-products including organs and offal (digestive tract) for human food should be kept separate from the carcass and other meat products and thoroughly cleaned with clean water.

2. Offal should have all the digestive food removed and disposed of in a barrel or an area away from the slaughter and processing area. The offal should be rinsed to remove all ingesta and checked for parasites. If parasites are found in the offal, it should be disposed of and not fed to any humans or animals.

3. To dispose of offal if infected with parasites, boil thoroughly and bury it, covering it with lime and dirt. Some offal, if approved by the health inspector, may be fed to animals after cooking thoroughly.

4. Hides should have a designated area for storage until further cleaned and readied for tanning. As soon as hides are removed, they should be placed in the designated area and kept dry. Dirt and hair from the hides should not be in the slaughter or processing area after the hides are removed from the animal.

Condemned Products

1. Parts of the carcass or parts of the internal organs that have been found to be diseased or not suitable for human food should be placed in a separate barrel or container away from the slaughter or processing area.

2. The condemned parts should be marked with a carbon powder or a blue ink so people will know it can not be used for human food.

3. Some condemned products can be used for animal food if approved by a health inspector for animal food. If approved, the condemned product should be boiled and kept separate from carcasses and other meat products until moving to be fed to animals.

4. Condemned products should not be fed to animals without first thoroughly cooking. Condemned products should not be given to people to eat. It can make people sick.

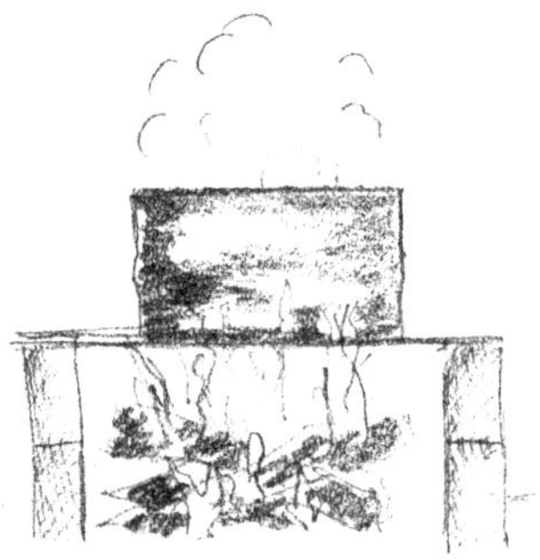

Boil by-products to be fed to animals.

Section VI

Pigs

Chapter 7
Pork Slaughter

Pork Slaughter

Psalms 24:1

The earth is the Lord's, and all it contains. The world, and those who dwell in it.

Restraining and Stunning

Hogs may be stunned by either a captive bolt or a rifle. The restraints that are available for hogs would include a small holding crate or a chute. The chute or crate must be in a position that the hog may be easily removed.

The hog may be hoisted with a chain or rope wrapped around one leg. If a crate is not available, have another person roll the hog over after stunning and keep it immobilized for bleeding.

The hog should be rolled onto its back and the person restraining the hog may place his feet on each side of the hog behind its shoulders. The forelegs should be held up straight and spread apart.

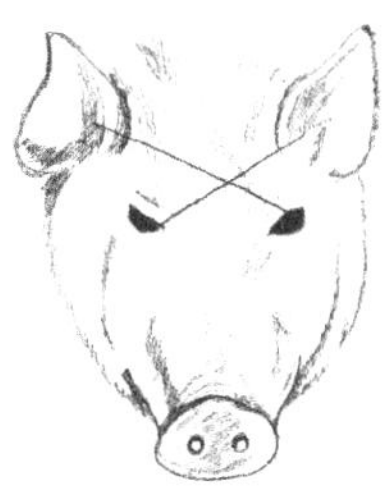

Middle of X to stun a hog.

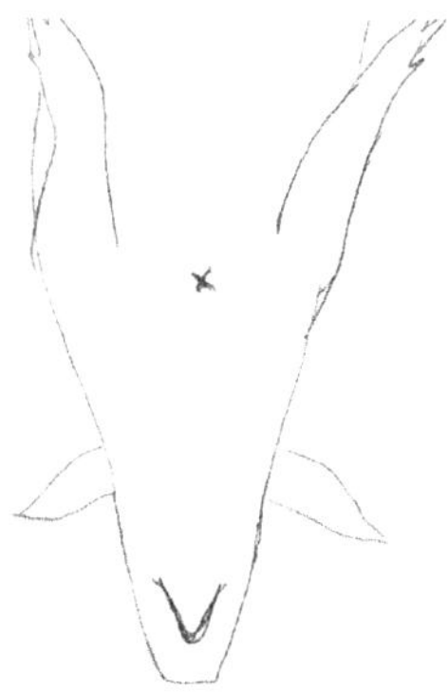

X marks area to stick a hog.

Bleeding

If the hog is hoisted with a chain or rope, one leg can be held with one hand and the other hand used to bleed the hog.

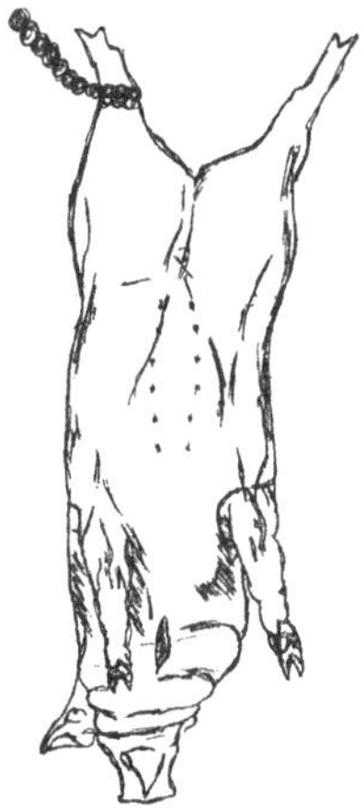

Hog hoisted that was bled.

Stick the knife blade, cutting edge up, straight in front of the breastbone (sternum). Then, the point of the knife should be directed between the breastbone (sternum) and the backbone and upwards toward the tail. This will sever the carotid arteries and jugular veins.

The knife should be withdrawn leaving a stick hole that should be not wider than the knife blade, to prevent any contamination from the scalding water. Do not stick the heart, allow the heart to beat the blood out of the body.

If the hog is restrained on the ground, stick the knife anterior to the sternum and the cutting edge towards the jaw. Go under the sternum at a 45° angle and push the blade of the knife up under the sternum and down. A gushing of blood should occur.

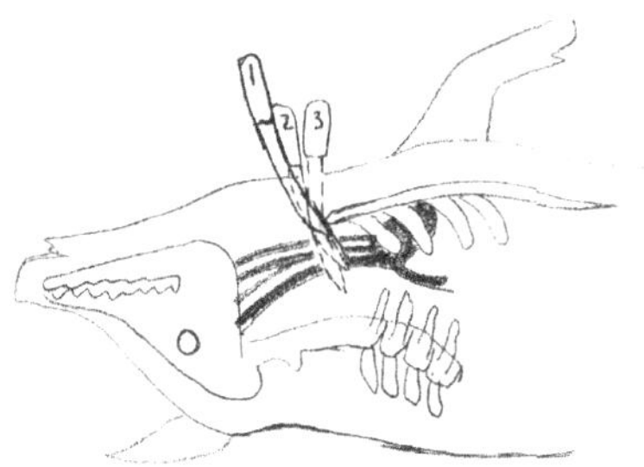

Knife motion to bleed.

Skinning a hog

For very large hogs, it may be easier to skin than to scald. To skin a hog, place the hog on its back in a cradle or skinning crate. If a cradle is not available, bricks or stones can be placed on each side of the hog to keep belly up.

To skin a hog, follow the same directions for skinning a beef. Remember that a hog has a thin skin that can be cut through easily. Keeping hands and knives clean during skinning is very important.

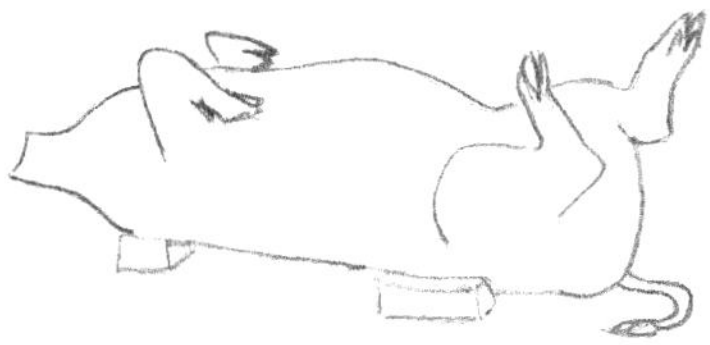

Hog propped with bricks for skinning.

Scalding

To scald a hog, a barrel or vat that is larger than the hog should be used. For very large hogs over 113 kilograms (250 pounds), it is recommended to skin the hog.

The barrel or vat should be placed below a platform, so the hog can be moved and placed in the container and then moved out. The temperature of the water should be between 61 plus or minus 1 degree C (143 plus or minus 2 degree F). A large vat may be used if it will hold enough water for the hog to stay immersed (below the water level).

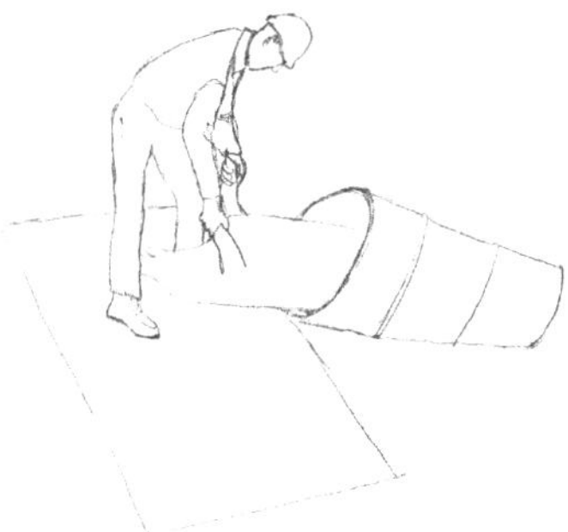

Placing hog into scalding barrel.

The temperature would allow an immersion time of 4 to 4 1/2 minutes. Overscalding will "set the hair" and also cook the skin, allowing contaminated scalding water to enter the meat. The lower the temperature, the more time that is required to scald the hog.

Keeping the barrel at an angle facilitates moving the hog in and out. A hook can be placed under the stunned and bled animal's jaw to move it to the vat.

The hog should be placed hind-end first into the barrel and continuously moved up and down until the hair loosens. The hair should be checked periodically during scalding.

The hind leg (ham), flank, belly, and head regions should be checked. Once the hair is determined to be loose, the hog should be immediately removed from the water.

Another method is to scald one-half of the hog at a time.

After the hind quarter has been scalded, the hog is removed and scraped and hind feet shaved so the tendons can be opened and a gambrel inserted into the hind legs.

The hog is then placed head first so the fore quarter can be scalded. After scalding the front end the hog may be scraped and shaved.

Hair Removal

After the hog is removed from the scalding vat, it should be immediately scraped using either bell scrapers or a knife.

The scrapers are designed to be held at an angle and pulled towards the person working the hair. When using a knife, keep the blade at an angle that it does not cut into the skin of the hog.

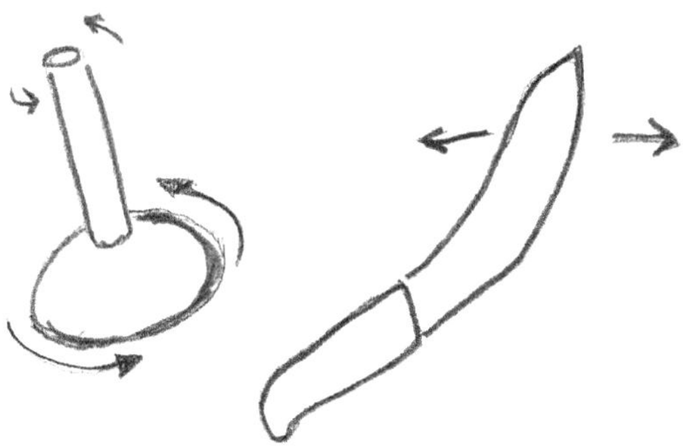

Back and forth motion with a bell scraper and a knife to remove hair.

A rapid movement back and forth with the scraper and the knife will remove the hair. Clean the hair thoroughly from around the legs and feet of the hog.

The head of the hog, if it is to be consumed, should be scraped around the head and the ears. The ears should be cleaned out of wax and dirt with a hook or a knife.

Trim the hair and skin surrounding the eye, including the eyelid, and the lips.

Remove the toenails and dewclaw nails with a hook. Hook under the nail and pull towards yourself, keeping clear of the hook.

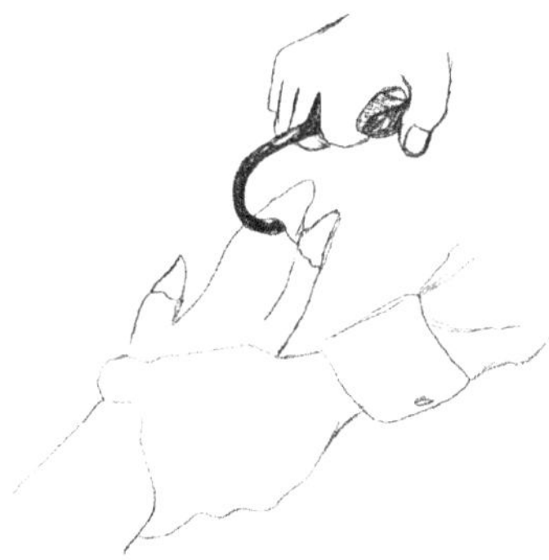

Pulling toenails with a hook.

Do not hold onto the leg of the carcass, as the hook could slip and hook into the person's arm.

The hind legs after being scraped should be rinsed off. A cut just above the dewclaws on the hind legs will expose the tendons that can be used to attach the hog to the gambrel. The hog should be rinsed after scraping and hoisted.

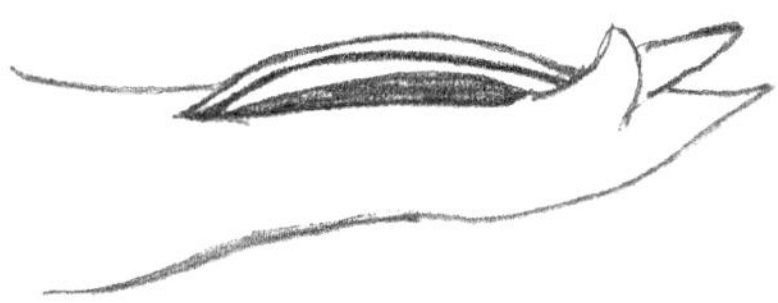

Exposed tendon for hanging on gambrel.

Head Removal

The head may be removed first before evisceration or after evisceration.

The head may be removed at the atlas joint with a knife or a saw. If the head meat and the tongue are desired, skin out the head and remove the head meat and the tongue.

Evisceration

To begin evisceration:

Open the breast bone (sternum) with a saw if a knife will not cut through the bone. This will open up the thoracic cavity to allow the lungs and heart (pluck) to come out easier. Be careful not to saw past the tip of the breastbone up into the heart.

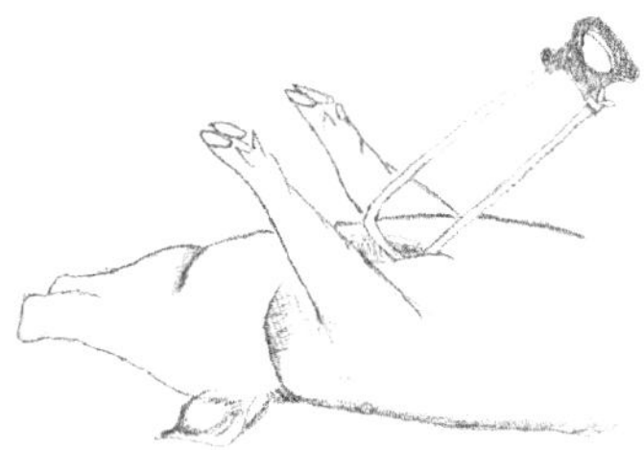

Opening breast bone for easier removal of lungs.

Cut around the bung and loosen it from its connective tissue. Tie off the bung with string and push it into the abdominal cavity.

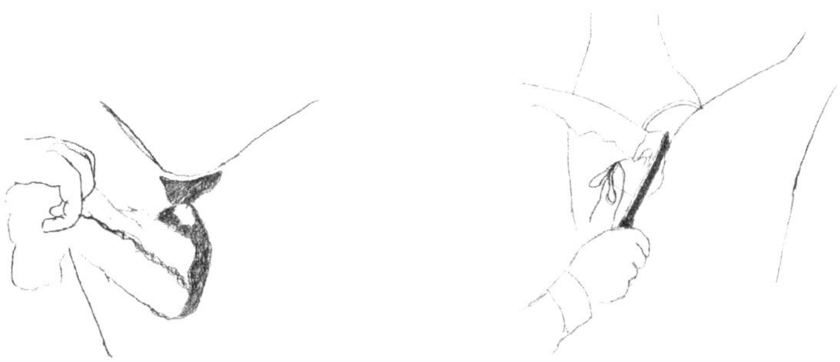

Loosening and tying bung.

On a male carcass, loosen the pizzle (penis) and remove it from the surface of the carcass and cut it loose at the pelvic junction. Open the pelvic region to cut the pizzle free from the pelvis.

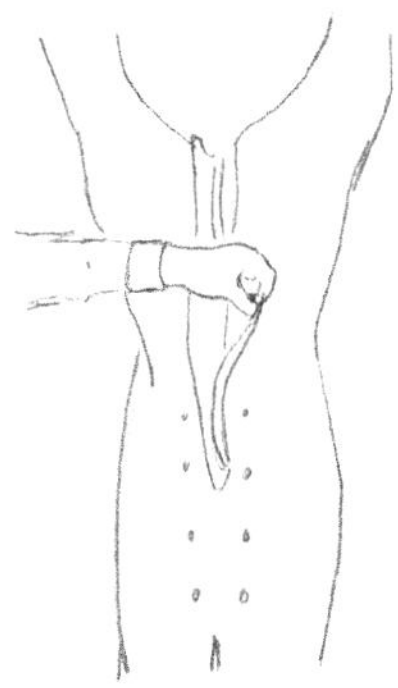

Removing the pizzle.

A saw cut through the pelvic bone, between the two hind legs will open the region and make it easier to remove the bung. Be careful not to cut down into the bung or the intestines.

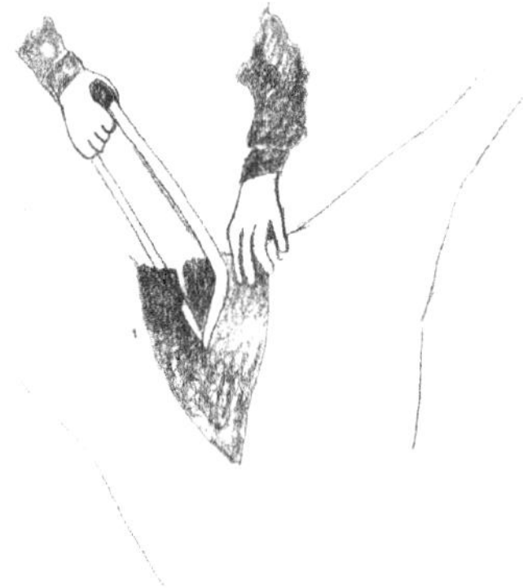

Sawing through pelvic bone.

Place the first two fingers of the hand into the opening of the abdomen to guard the knife point. The knife handle may also be turned inside the carcass with the blade pointing down and the tip out.

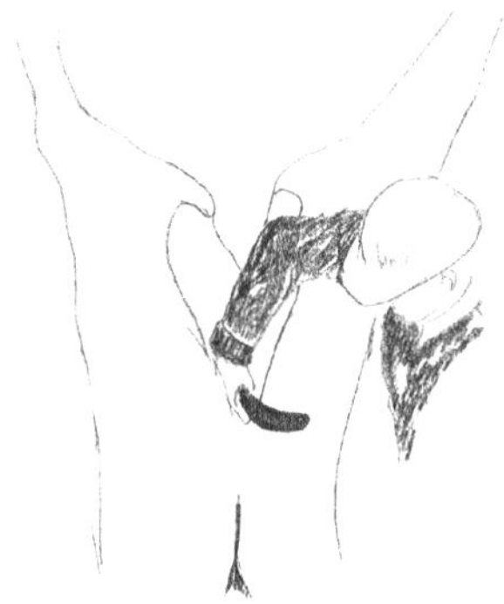

Opening abdomen.

Carefully open the midline of the carcass down to the point were the breast was opened. Pull the bung outward from the carcass. Remove the bladder and continue cutting the tissue behind the intestinal tract to separate it from the body wall.

Be careful that the intestinal tract is not ruptured. The intestines and stomach should all roll out of the carcass as it is being pushed down.

The liver may be removed with the abdominal tract, and the gall bladder removed from the liver.

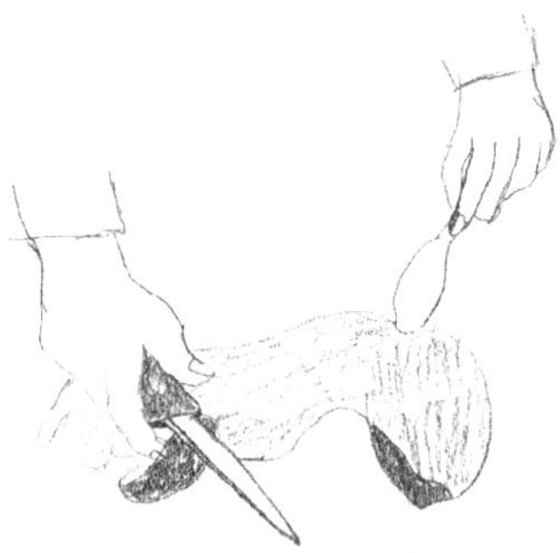

Removing gallbladder from liver.

The pluck (lungs and heart) may next be removed after cutting around the diaphragm muscle to expose the thoracic cavity. Or the pluck (lungs and heart) may come out with all of the internal organs, and then removed from the esophagus (food tube) and rest of the organs.

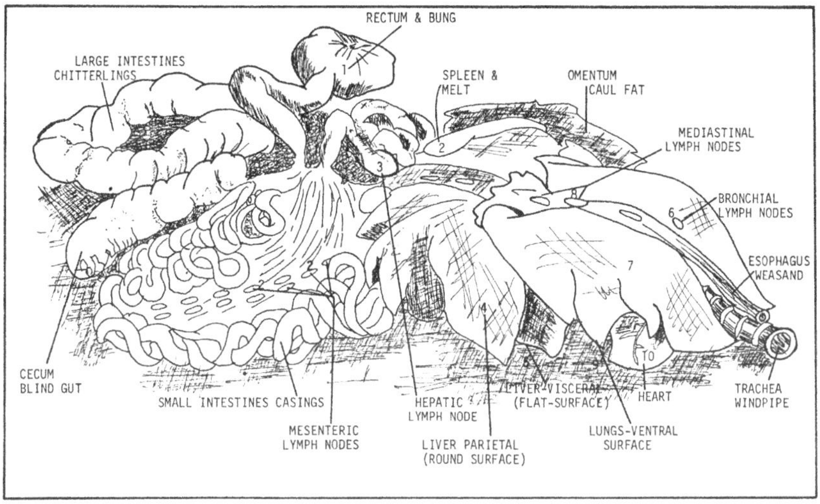

Internal organs of hog with lymph nodes.
(USDA 1977)

Wash the inside and outside of the carcass. Wash thoroughly down the inside of the neck and trim any excess blood if necessary.

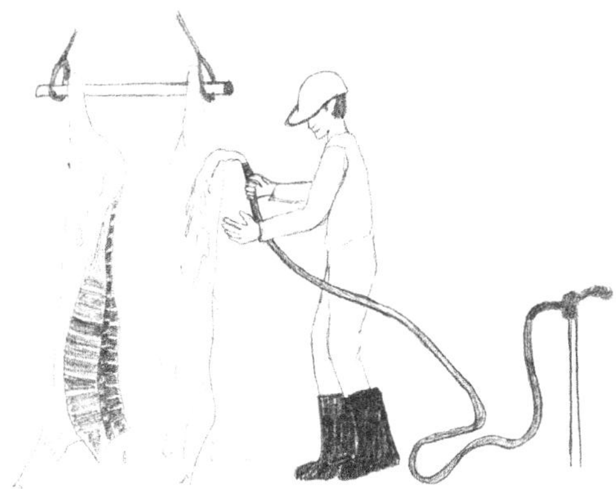

Washing carcass inside and out.

By-products and skins

By-products including organs and offal (digestive tract) for human food should be kept separate from the carcass and other meat products and thoroughly washed inside and outside with clean water.

Offal should have all the animal's digestion food (ingesta) removed and disposed of in a barrel or an area away from the slaughter and processing area. The offal should be washed to remove all ingesta and checked for parasites. If parasites are found in the offal, it should be disposed of and not fed to any humans or animals.

To dispose of offal infected with parasites, boil it thoroughly and then bury it, covering it with lime and dirt. Some offal, if approved by the health inspector, may be fed to animals after cooking thoroughly.

Skins should have a designated area for storage until further processing for tanning. As soon as a skin is removed, it should be placed in the designated area and kept dry. Dirt and hair from the skins should not be in the slaughter or processing area after the skins or hair is removed from the animal.

Condemned Products

Parts of the carcass and/or parts of the internal organs that are diseased or "not suitable for human food" should be placed in a separate barrel or container away from the slaughter or processing area. This barrel should be marked to indicate the contents.

The condemned parts should be marked with a carbon powder or a blue ink so people will know it can not be used for human food.

Some condemned products can be used for animal food if approved by a health inspector. If approved, the condemned product should be boiled and kept separate from human food until moved to be fed to animals.

Condemned products should not be fed to animals without first thoroughly cooking. Condemned products should not be given to people to eat. It can make people sick.

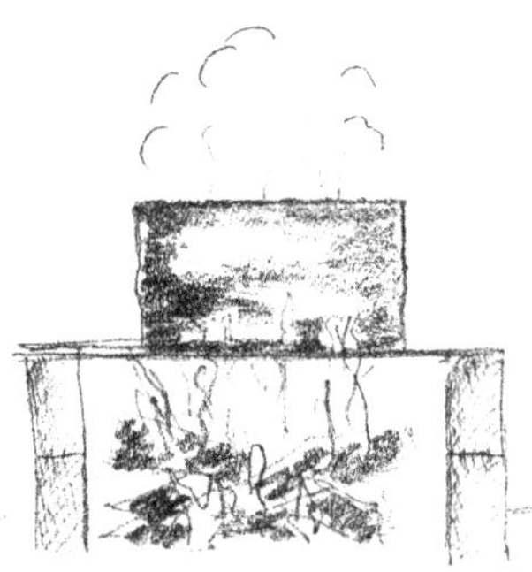

Boil by-products to be fed to animals.

Section VII

Sheep, Goats and Small Ruminants

Chapter 8

Sheep and Lamb Slaughter

Sheep and Lamb Slaughter

PROVERBS 27:26-27

The lambs will be for your clothing, and the goats will bring the price of a field.

And there will be goats' milk enough for your food, for the food of your household, and sustenance for your maidens.

Handling of sheep and lambs is important to prevent bruising of the carcass. Pulling the live animal with the fleece will cause bruising. Sheep should not be handled by the legs, but should be lead with one hand under the jaw and the other hand behind the dock.

Sheep should be fasted up to 24 hours prior to slaughter but still given a good water supply. The fasting will also allow removal of the pelt easier.

Keeping tools and hands clean at all times is very important for the overall cleanliness of the carcass. The fell is a colorless, thin membrane found just below the pelt (fleece). The fell separates the pelt from the carcass and should be kept intact because it helps prevent drying out of the carcass.

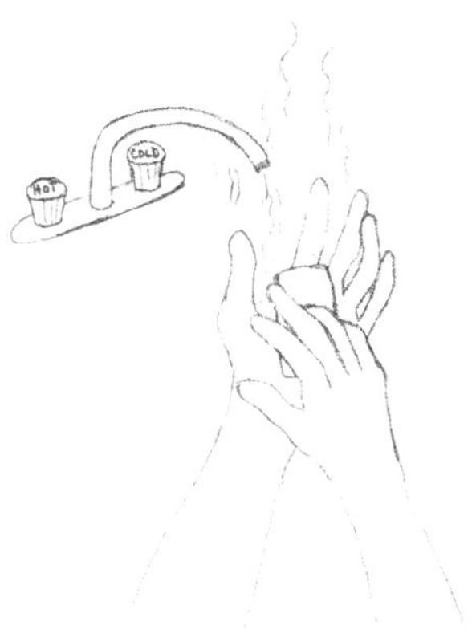

Keep hands very clean when slaughtering sheep.

Stunning and Bleeding

The lamb or sheep may be stunned with a sharp blow on top of the head if they do not have horns. A rifle may be used to stun in the same area between the ears and eyes as cattle and hogs.

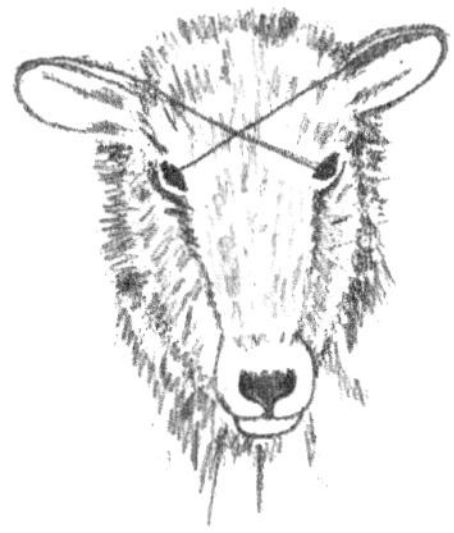

Middle of X to stun a sheep.

Either method may be used effectively depending on the size of the lamb or sheep. To be bled, the animal may be hoisted with a chain or rope or placed on a cradle or rack.

Holding the ear or jaw, place the knife behind the jaw, with the blade edge outward. The knife point can be inserted past the other jaw and pulled straight outward severing the jugular veins and the carotid arteries.

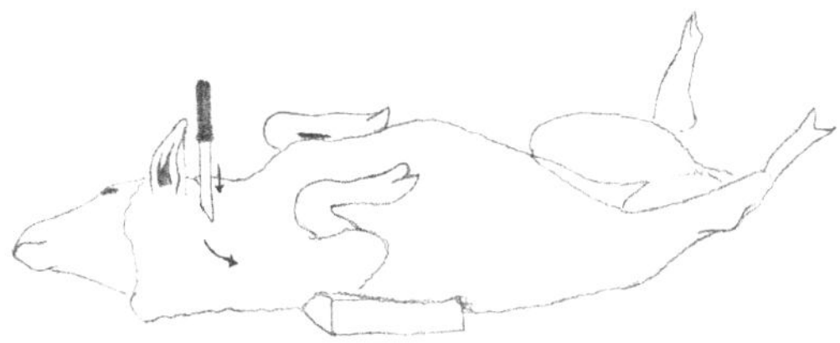

Bleeding by placing knife behind the jaw and cutting outward.

Pelting

Utilizing a cradle or rack, place the lamb on its back and open the pelt down the front of each foreleg from the break joint to the breast.

The two cuts should meet in a point in front of the breast. The forelegs should be skinned out, taking care to prevent the pelt from coming back up on the legs and keeping hands and knives clean.

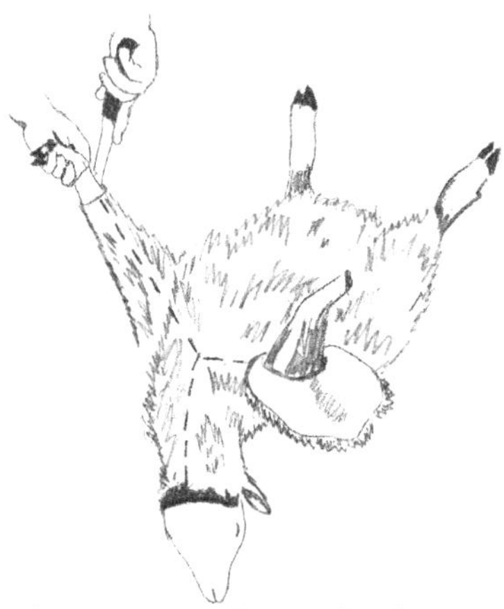

Removing the hooves and opening fleece down legs.

The front leg should be removed at the break joint at the cannon bone just above the hock. In young lambs, this will be easily removed by twisting the lower leg. In mutton (older sheep) this joint will not be easily broken and a knife will have to be used to remove the hoof.

The hind leg should be opened down the back from the hoof to the bung. Keep the knife blade close to the pelt when making this cut to prevent cutting into the fell (the membrane that is under the pelt) or cutting into the muscle.

Remove the foot at the joint with the hoof. Again, making sure that hands and knives are kept clean.

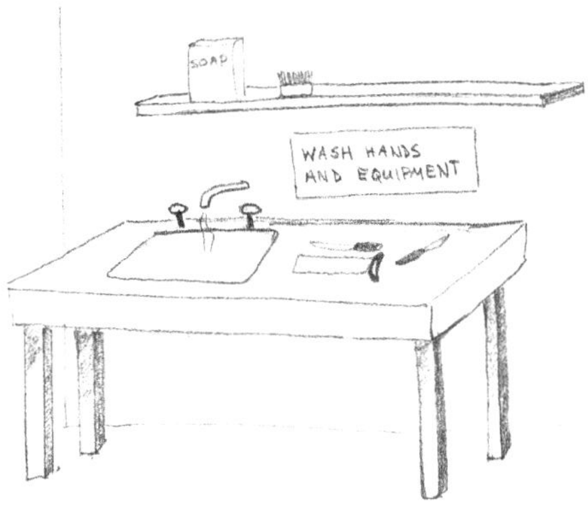

Keep hands and all equipment clean.

Using the fist of one hand begin to work up under the pelt at the flank region. Use the other hand to pull the pelt up as the fisting process takes place.

Fist up over the flank. From the direction of the breast, begin fisting up over the breast and over the belly. Fist towards the pelt, and try not to fist down towards the carcass.

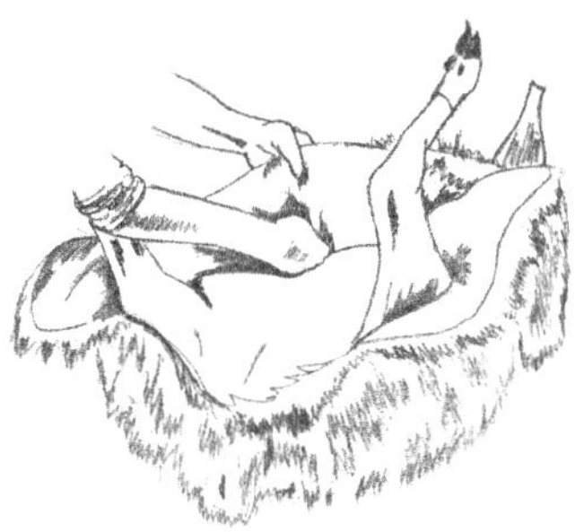

"Fisting" to remove fleece.

Continue fisting down the sides until the pelt is loosened down the front of the carcass.

The carcass may be hoisted at this point for ease in final fisting and evisceration.

The end of the esophagus should be securely tied with string to prevent contents of the stomach from coming out during evisceration. The trachea (windpipe) and esophagus (food tube) can be separated with a weasand rod. If this is not possible, hold one end of the esophagus and move your hand up the esophagus to separate the connective tissue between the trachea and the esophagus.

With the lamb still lying on the rack, open the breast bone with a saw. Tie the tendons of both hind legs together, and insert with hook to hang or hoist the lamb.

Open the midline of the pelt and continue fisting the pelt towards the back. Fist up the back leg to avoid breaking the fell. Continue fisting until the pelt has been loosened and is hanging down around the head.

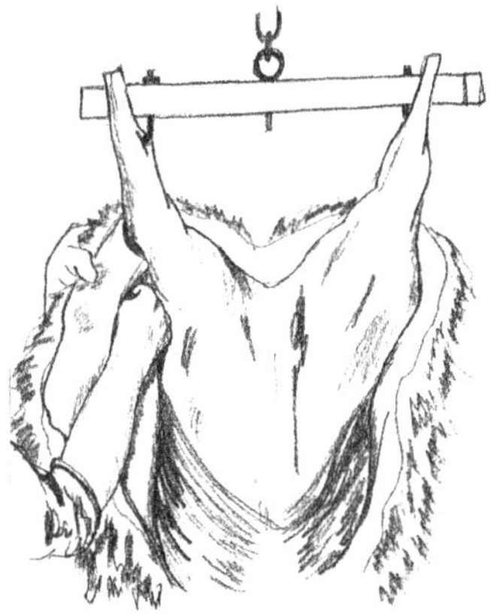

"Fisting" around hind legs.

Do not allow the pelt to fall back on the carcass and contaminate the carcass. At this point the head may be removed at the atlas joint with a knife or a saw. If the head meat and the tongue are desired off the lamb, skin out the head and remove the head meat and the tongue.

Evisceration

Cut around the bung and loosen it from its connective tissue. Tie off the bung with string and push it into the abdominal cavity.

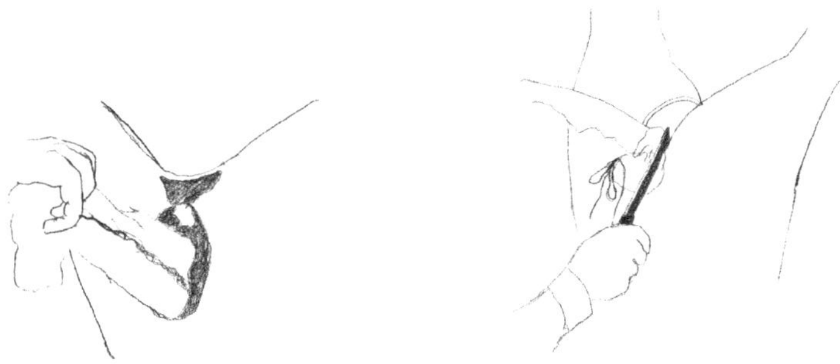

Loosening and tying bung.

On a male carcass, loosen the pizzle (penis) and remove it from the surface of the carcass and cut it loose at the pelvic junction. Open the cod into the pelvic region to cut the pizzle free from the pelvis.

Place the first two fingers of the hand into the opening of the abdomen to guard the knife point. The knife handle may also be turned inside the carcass with the blade pointing down and the tip out.

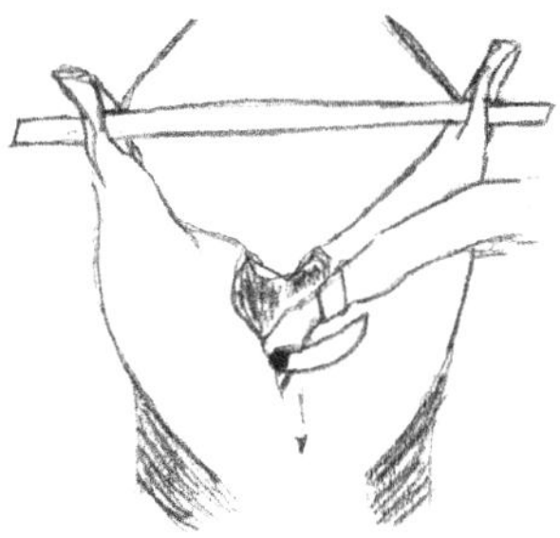

Knife pointing outward and downward during evisceration.

Carefully open the midline of the carcass down to the point where the breast was opened. Pull the bung outward from the carcass. Remove the bladder and continue cutting the tissue behind the intestinal tract to separate it from the body wall. Be careful that the intestinal tract is not ruptured.

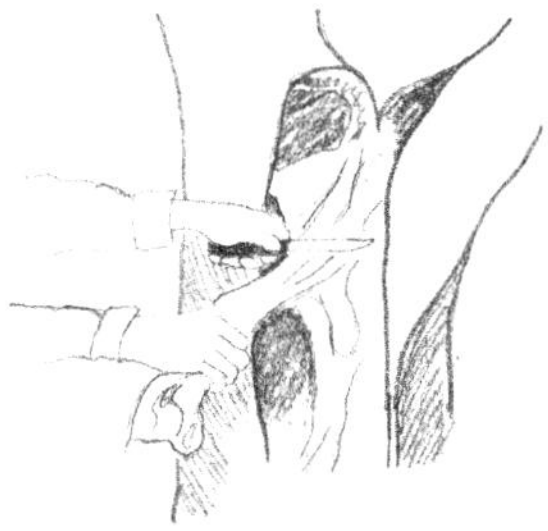

Removing intestines carefully.

The intestines and rumen should all roll out of the carcass as it is being pushed down.

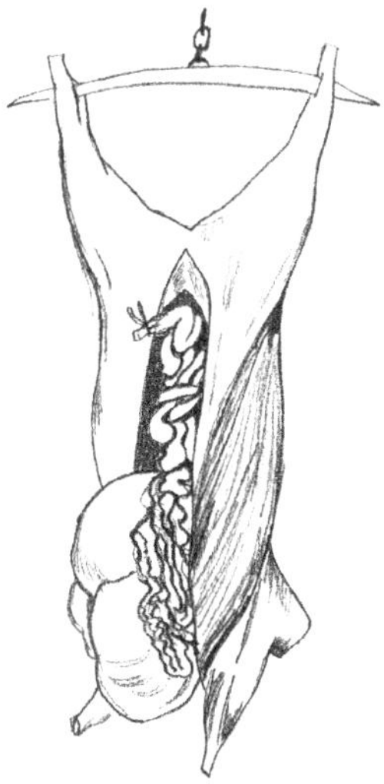

Carcass with bung tied and pulled loose with rumen out.

The liver may be removed with the abdominal tract, and the gall bladder removed from the liver. The pluck (lungs and heart) may next be removed after cutting around the diaphragm muscle to expose the thoracic cavity.

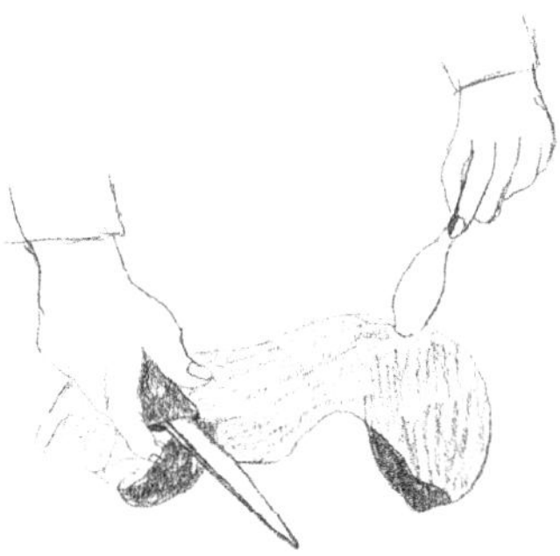

Removing gall bladder from liver.

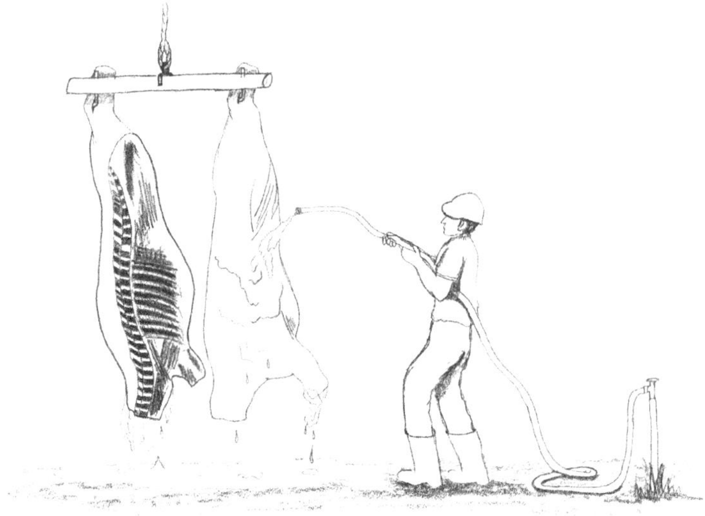

Washing carcass inside and out.

Wash the inside and outside of the carcass. Wash thoroughly down the inside of the neck and trim any excess blood if necessary.

Double the fore shank up against the forearm and find the tendon in the forearm. Use this tendon to anchor the fore shank up against the forearm. This keeps the fore shank from becoming dirty when moving the carcass and further processing.

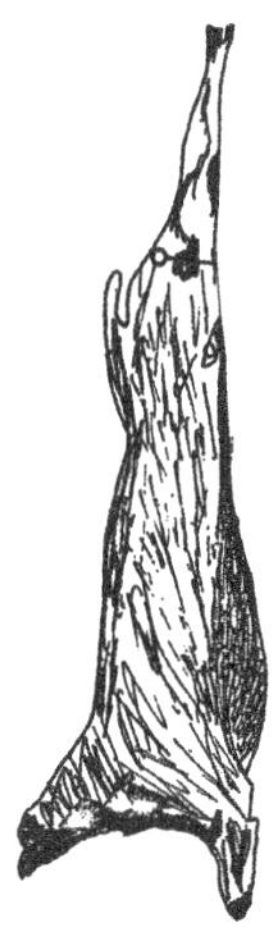

Lamb carcass with forelegs tied up.

By-products and pelts and skins

By-products including organs and offal (digestive tract) for human food should be kept separate from the carcass and other meat products and thoroughly washed inside and outside with clean water.

Offal should have all the animal's digestion food (ingesta) removed and disposed of in a barrel or an area away from the slaughter and processing area. The offal should be washed to remove all ingesta and checked for parasites. If parasites are found in the offal, it should be disposed of and not fed to any humans or animals.

To dispose of offal infected with parasites, boil it thoroughly and then bury it, covering it with lime and dirt. Some offal, if approved by the health inspector, may be fed to animals after cooking thoroughly.

Skins and fleeces should have a designated area for storage until further processing for tanning. As soon as a skin and fleece is removed, it should be placed in the designated area and kept dry. Dirt and hair from the hides should not be in the slaughter or processing area after the skins or fleeces are removed from the animal.

Condemned Products

Parts of the carcass and/or parts of the internal organs that are diseased or "not suitable for human food" should be placed in a separate barrel or container away from the slaughter or processing area. This barrel should be marked to indicate the contents.

The condemned parts should be marked with a carbon powder or a blue ink so people will know it can not be used for human food.

Some condemned products can be used for animal food if approved by a health inspector for animal food. If approved, the condemned product should be boiled and kept separate from human food until moved to be fed to animals.

Condemned products should not be fed to animals without first thoroughly cooking. Condemned products should not be given to people to eat. It can make people sick.

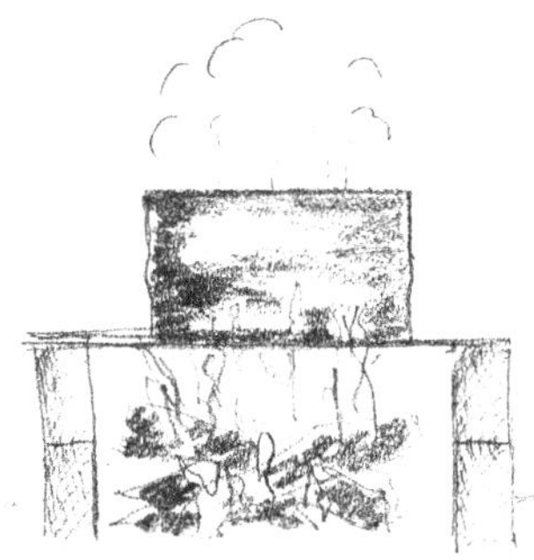

Boil by-products to be fed to animals.

Chapter 9

Slaughtering of Other Small Ruminants—Goats, Antelope, Deer

Slaughtering of Other Small Ruminants—Goats, Antelope, Deer

PROVERBS 12:10

A righteous man has regard for the life of his beast, but the compassion of the wicked is cruel.

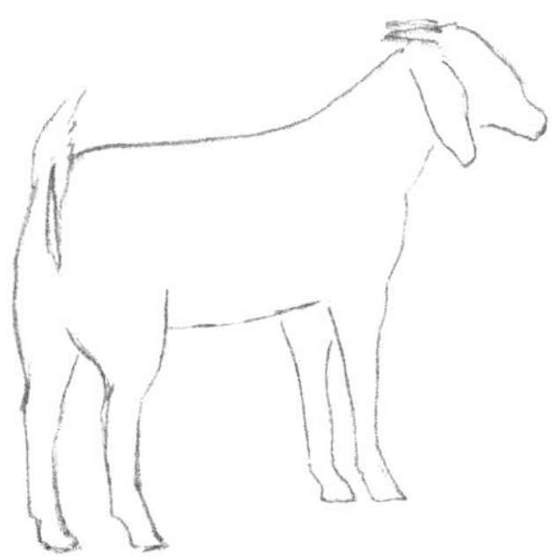

Goats, antelope, deer and other small ruminants can be slaughtered very similar to sheep. Follow the procedures for sheep slaughter. However, with goats and antelopes, skinning may be done with a knife since they do not have a fleece. Continue to keep the hands and knives very clean.

Remove the hooves and skin and move it to other areas away from the skinned carcass to prevent cross-contamination.

Tie off the bung and place it back into the abdominal cavity.

When removing the internal organs, pull the bung out towards the worker to prevent contamination of the carcass.

Remove the bladder sac and then begin to pull the intestines out.

The rumen (large stomach) should come out easily. Be careful not to puncture the intestines or the rumen.

The esophagus (food tube) will still be attached to the trachea (windpipe) of the lungs. The lungs and heart (pluck) may be removed still attached to the digestive tract and then cut loose from the digestive tract for further inspection.

The guidelines for by-products, skins and condemned products are the same as mentioned in the sheep and lamb slaughter.

Section VIII

Poultry and Small Animals

Chapter 10

Poultry Slaughter and Processing

Poultry Slaughter and Processing

Matthew 6:25-26

For this reason I (God) say to you, do not be anxious for your life, as to what you shall eat, or what you shall drink; nor for your body, as to what you shall put on. Is not life more than food, and the body than clothing?

Look at the birds of the air, that they do not sow, neither do they reap, nor gather into barns, and yet your heavenly Father feeds them. Are you not worth much more than they?

Slaughtering Chickens

1. Chickens should be kept off feed for 24 hour prior to slaughter. This will clean the digestive tract and make it cleaner during evisceration. They should have free access to water.

2. Chickens should be hung with strong twine or wire from a convenient height for working.

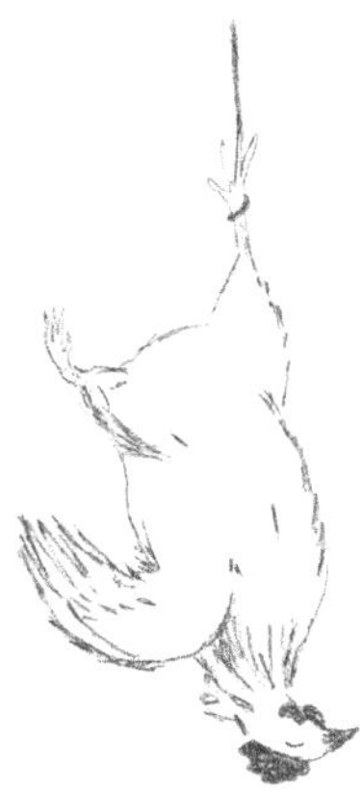

Hanging a chicken.

3. A blood cup, a can weighted at the bottom, can be hooked to the mandible of the chicken to catch the blood. The weight prevents the chicken from moving around too much.

4. Hang a chicken by its legs and hold the head with the comb with one hand. Insert the knife into the groove in the roof of the mouth of the bird and force the knife into the rear part of the skull, going into the brain. This stuns the bird.

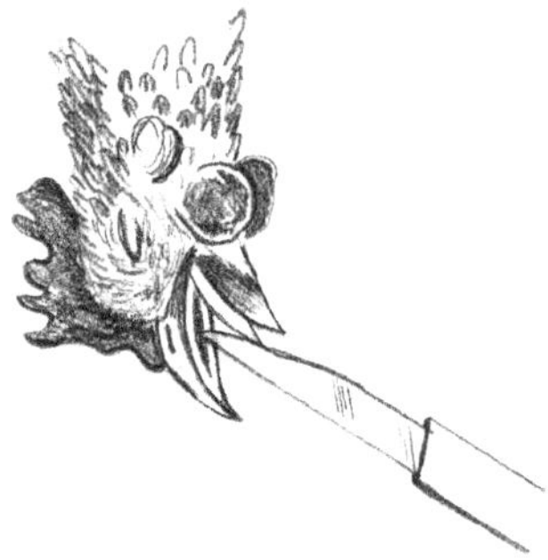

Inserting knife into mouth.

Then insert the knife back into one side of the throat and cut to the opposite side and pull the knife out. Allow all the blood to drain out into the cup.

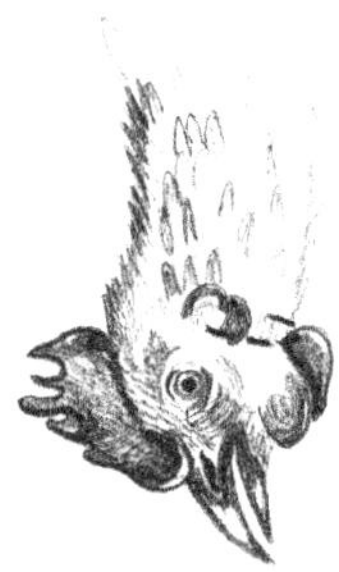

Cut outward to bleed.

Dry Picking

1. Chickens may be dry picked if only a few chickens are being prepared.
2. As soon as the bird is dead, begin picking in the direction in which the feathers lie.
3. Begin with the feathers over the breast, picking a few so as not to tear the skin.

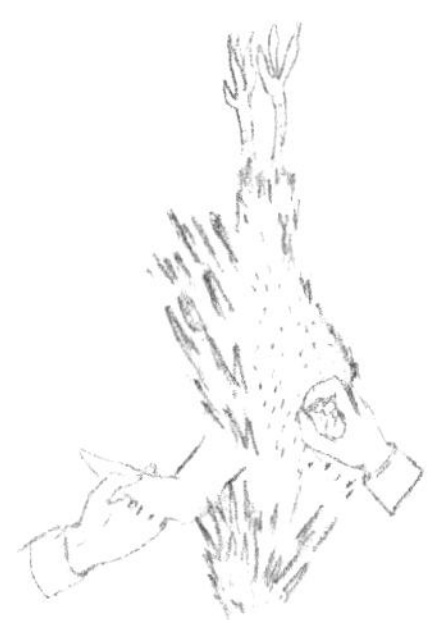

Plucking feathers from breast.

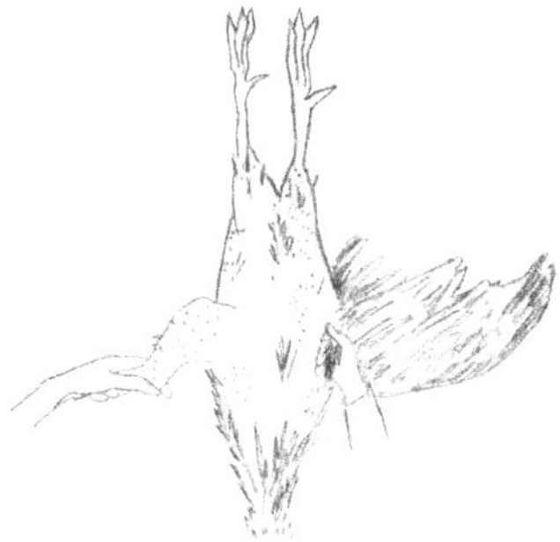

Plucking feathers from wings.

4. Next do the neck and the body, finishing up with the wings and tail.

Wet Picking

1. Dip the dead birds one at a time into water at approximately 53° C , plus or minus 2 degrees (128° F or minus 2 degrees) for 30 seconds.

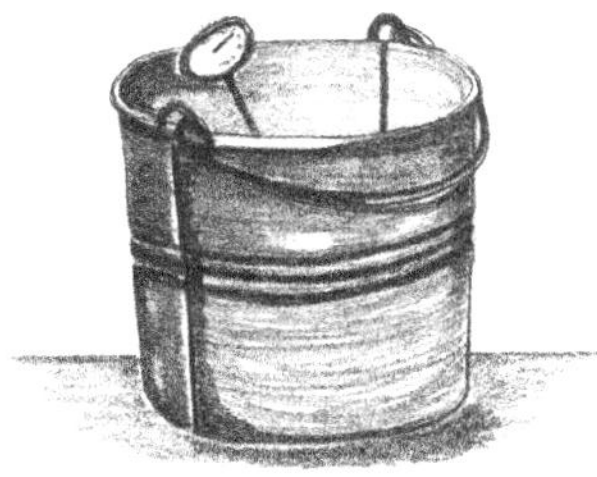

Check temperature of water.

2. Continue to move the bird up and down in the water to soak through the feathers onto the skin. Adding some soap to the water will allow the water to get past the oil in the feathers of duck and geese.

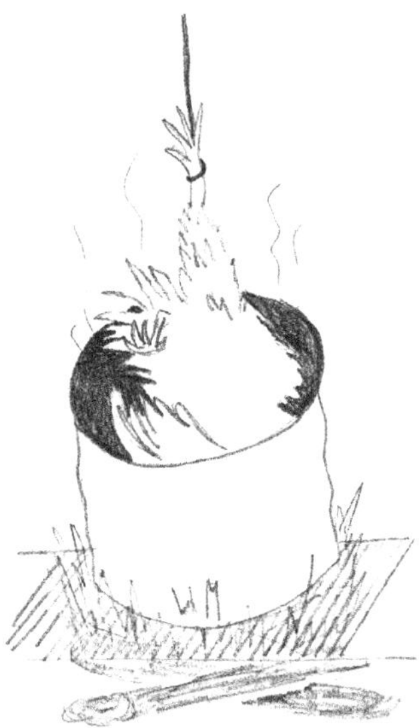

Soaking bird in hot water.

3. Do not soak the bird too long in the hot water, because it could cook the skin underneath.

4. Pinfeathers come out easier with cool water. The pinfeathers can even be rubbed out or removed with a knife pulling across the feather or with tweezers.

5. Any hair may be singed with a small flame or a propane torch.

6. The legs and head should be scrubbed with a stiff brush.

7. Rinse the carcass with cool water.

Dressing the Bird

1. Remove the head at the joint between the head and neck.

2. Remove the oil gland on the back just in front of the tail.

3. Cut from in front of the nipple of the oil sack toward the rear and scoop out all of the oil gland.

4. Cut the feet off at the hock.

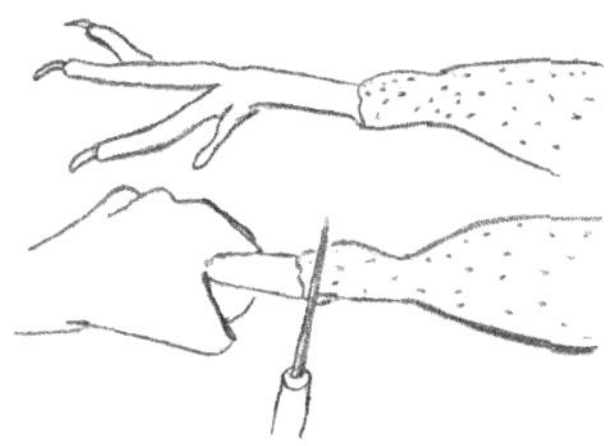

Remove feet at hock.

5. Place the bird on its back, begin to cut through the skin at the shoulder, and cut up the back of the neck, peeling back the skin to where the head was removed.

6. Using the tip of the knife move it back and forth to slip between two vertebrae and twist. This will remove the neck from the body.

7. Remove the crop (large pouch), windpipe, and gullet.

8. The crop can be removed by hooking the gullet between the crop and gizzard with a hook or a finger, then pull the crop loose from the skin.

9. Make a cut under the rear of the breastbone.

10. Cut down and around the anus and the tail and back up, be careful not to cut the intestines.

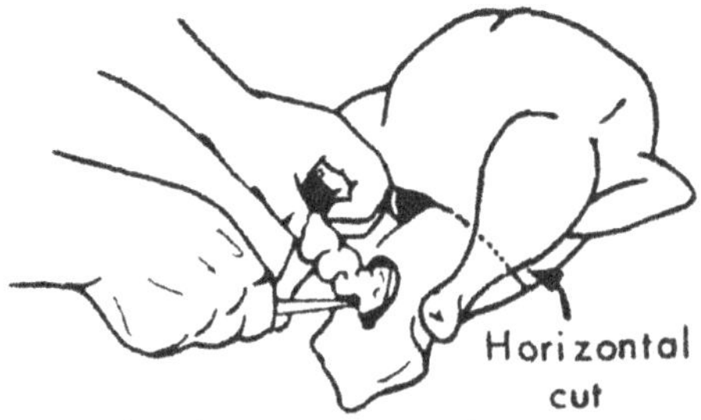

Cut down and around anus.

11. Hold the anus and with the other hand, go up under the breastbone and scoop the insides out.

12. The gizzard may require going back in to remove it.

13. Remove the liver and trim out the gall bladder

14. Trim the heart and wash it.

15. Cut the gizzard through its side and peel out its lining.

16. Chill the gizzard, heart, liver and neck.

17. Remove the gonads (testicles) from up under the back.

18. Scrape out the lungs with a hook or a finger.

19. Rinse the carcass inside and out with clean water not used on another carcass.

20. Allow the body heat to escape by allowing cool running water to flow over the bird in a container.

21. The carcasses may also be placed in a tub of ice to chill

22. Keep the carcasses below 1.4° C (40° F) or lower.

23. Pull the carcasses from the tube of ice and allow to drain before wrapping.

24. Dry the bird and place it in a plastic or waterproof sack.

25. The bird may be wrapped and frozen or kept chilled.

Cutting up the Bird

Quartering a Chicken

1. Place the chicken on the back, and cut in half along the breast bone.

2. This takes a sharp knife, so be careful in holding the chicken to make this cut.

3. Pull the two sections apart and break the ribs away from the backbone and finish cutting with the knife.

4. Take each half and separate the leg-thigh combination from the breast-wing portion by cutting between the thigh and the breast.

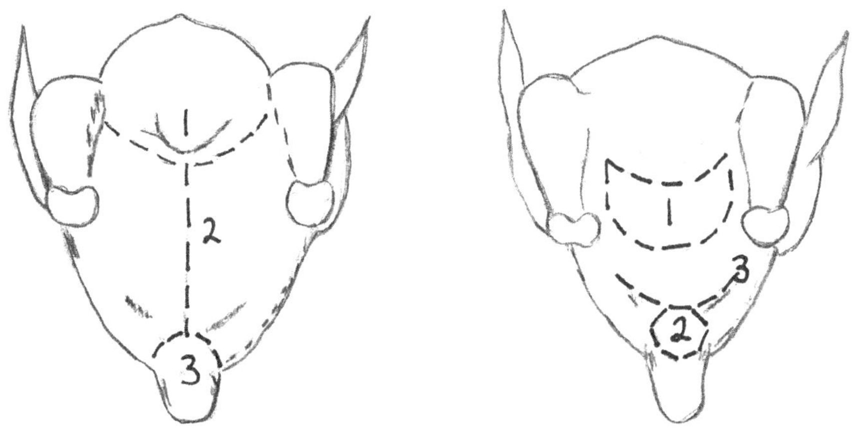

Two ways to cut up poultry.

Turkeys

1. Turkeys should be picked utilizing hotter water than chickens.

2. Dry picking may also be desirable.

3. Wash the bird thoroughly with cool water.

4. Turkeys should be allowed to cool for 24 hours before freezing.

5. Turkeys may be cooked whole or cut into larger cuts by removing the legs, wings and breast.

Ducks and Geese

1. Dry picking works best with ducks and geese because of the water-resistant feathers and down.

2. Feathers should be pulled downward in the direction that they grow.

3. Pulling upward will cause the skin to tear.

4. To remove feathers form the breast, the feathers should be picked close to the skin and rolled outwardly.

5. This will remove the feathers neatly.

6. Pluck row after row of feathers to leave an undamaged skin.

7. Paraffin (hot wax) may be used on ducks and geese after they have been picked to remove excess feathers.

8. The bird should be chilled before dipping in paraffin.

9. The bird should be dipped for 5 to 10 seconds and then hung to cool for 2 minutes.

10. The paraffin should cool over the carcass. Pull the paraffin off.

11. Wash the bird thoroughly in cool water to chill the carcass.

Chapter 11

Rabbits and Other Small Animal Slaughter

Rabbits and Other Small Animals

PSALMS 136:24-25

Who (God) remembered us in our low estate, for His loving kindness is everlasting, and has rescued us from our adversaries, for His loving kindness is everlasting.

Who gives food to all flesh, for His loving kindness is everlasting.

Young rabbits from 2 to 6 months old have the most desirable meat. Older rabbits may be utilized as roasters.

Slaughter and Skinning Rabbits

Killing a rabbit is fairly simple. Hold the hind legs and hit it behind the ears on the neck with a club. If the rabbit is too large, another person can hold the rabbit behind the shoulders and hold the ears over the face. Another person can then stun with the club. The head should be removed immediately with a sharp knife to completely bleed out the blood.

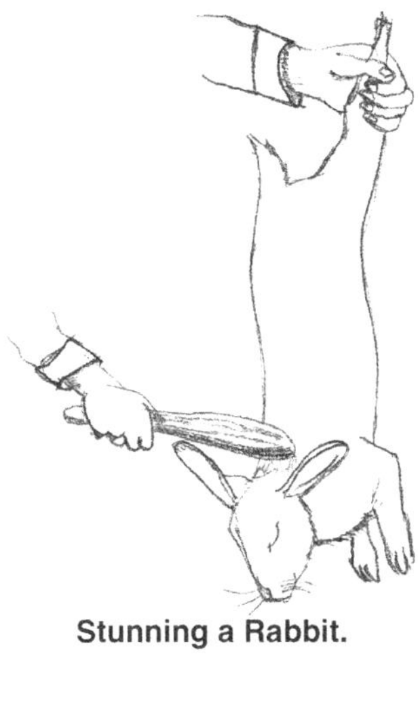

Stunning a Rabbit.

Hang the rabbit by one gambrel (hind hock) joint on a screw hook or a nail on a beam. The beam should be at a height that is comfortable to work. Remove the hock of the other rear leg at the hock joint, and the front feet and the tail.

Skin the free leg back to the anus with your fingers. A knife should only be used to begin the skinning process. Skin the other leg (the one that is hooked on the beam) down to the anus, without using the knife. Then peel the whole hide down and over the body.

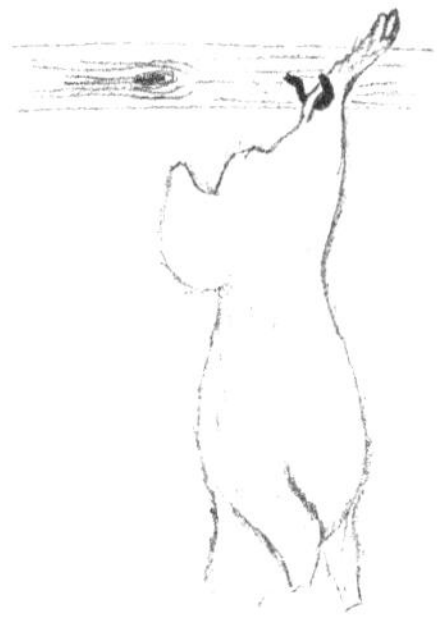

Hanging carcass to skin.

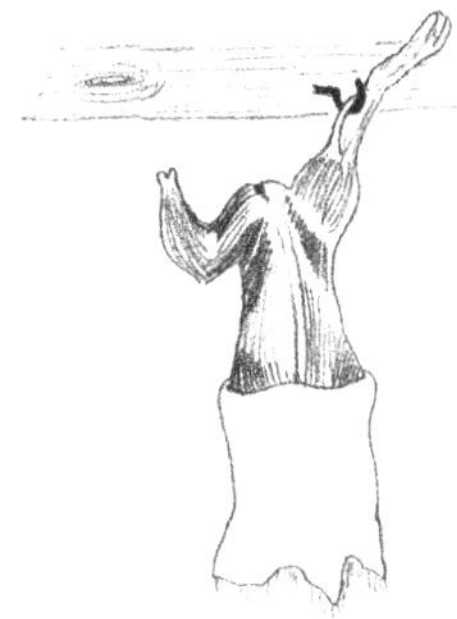

Legs skinned and peeling hide.

Make a slit down the midline of the rabbit, the full length of the body from the anus to the front of the sternum (breastbone), being careful not to puncture the intestines while removing the viscera. Some leave the liver, kidneys, and heart in. It is not advisable to leave the organs in the carcass.

Immediately rinse the carcass in cool water.

Processing the Rabbit

Rabbits and small animals may be cut into seven pieces: two hind legs, two loins, two front legs and the back or into nine pieces: two front legs, two hind legs, tail back, two ribs and two shoulder pieces as shown below.

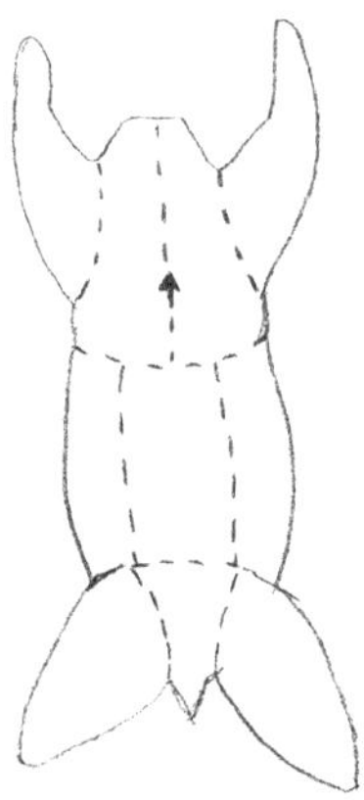

Cutting pattern on rabbit.

1. Hind Legs:
   Cut straight up beside the tail on each side.
   Cut beside the backbone until the knife reaches the hip joint at each leg.
   The hip joint can be cut through to remove the hind legs from the back.
   The tail can be removed by cutting down from the backbone beginning at the top of the tail.
2. Two Loins
   Remove Back and Flanks
   Cut across the backbone behind the ribs to remove the back from the rib (fore quarter of the carcass).
   The flanks can be cut from the back.
   The backbone can be split down the middle.

3. Follow the natural seam between the foreleg and the ribs to remove the front legs.
4. Remove the ribs in one piece by cutting through the top of the ribs, beside the backbone.
5. Wash the rabbit meat in cool water. Wrap and freeze.

Other Small Animals

Other small animals including guinea pigs, woodchucks, and local wild animals may be prepared in the same method as rabbits. Some animal pelts may not be as easily pulled as a rabbit. If this is the case then the animal may be carefully skinned.

Depending upon the size of the animal, the carcass may be cut into seven pieces or into only two pieces, the hind and forequarters or left whole.

A whole carcass may be allowed to dry in the sun on a rack. Open up the carcass and stretch open the thoracic and abdominal cavity by cutting one side of the ribs. Sticks may be placed inside the carcass to stretch it open to facilitate drying.

Section IX

Preservation and Storage

Chapter 12

Preservation of Meat

Preservation of Meat

MATTHEW 5:13-14

You are the salt of the earth, but if salt has lost its taste (its strength, its quality), how can its saltiness be restored? It is not good for anything any longer but to be thrown out and trodden underfoot by men. You are the light of the world. A city set on a hill cannot be hidden.

If meat cannot be eaten quickly, it should be preserved in some way to prevent germs (bacteria) from spoiling the meat. Meat that is not preserved can make humans sick. There are many ways to preserve meat, with and without cooling.

Boiling Meat for Further Usage

1. Meat can be cut immediately after slaughter into thin threadlike strips. The strips are wrapped around long sticks and allowed to dry and can also to be stored on the stick.

2. Boil the meat with fat. Next roast the meat, dry and crush the meat into pieces then mix with suitable fat and then store.

3. Pieces of meat can be cut, boiled in fat and removed from the boiling pot. The meat may then be placed in skin bags and stored for long periods of time without spoiling.

4. During dry seasons, meat may be loosely wrapped in a material that allows water to pass through, such as burlap material, and placed in a cool, high place for storage. The storage area should be dry and dark. Some groups of people utilize the thatched shelving in a darkened area for storage. It is difficult to store meat during rainy seasons.

5. Meat may be boiled in water to remove excess blood and bacteria. This will allow the meat to be stored longer without spoiling under normal conditions.

6. If to be consumed quickly, meat may be stored in a cool area suspended in air for no more than three days.

Drying of Meat

1. Traditionally meat has been dried either over an open flame or in the sun.

2. Meat to be dried should be cut in thin strips for faster drying.

3. The best method to dry meat is in an oven. The oven may be kept at a low temperature to allow slow drying of the meat.

4. Drying of meat removes as much water as possible from the surface and the inside of the meat. Removal of water, necessary for microbial growth, allows the meat to be stored for longer periods of time.

5. Dried meat should be stored in an air-tight container, either a jar with a screw lid or in a sealed plastic bag. This will prevent any mold formation.

Salting of Meat

1. Salting is an old method to preserve meat and has been used for centuries

2. If salt is plentiful, it is an effective way to preserve meat.

3. Salt will not kill all the microorganisms (germs) and parasites.

4. Salted foods must be completely cooked to be made safe.

5. Use either a clean plastic or wooden container to salt meat in.

6. Approximately 16 kilograms (35 pounds) of salt for each 45 kilograms (100 pounds) kilograms of raw meat will be needed.

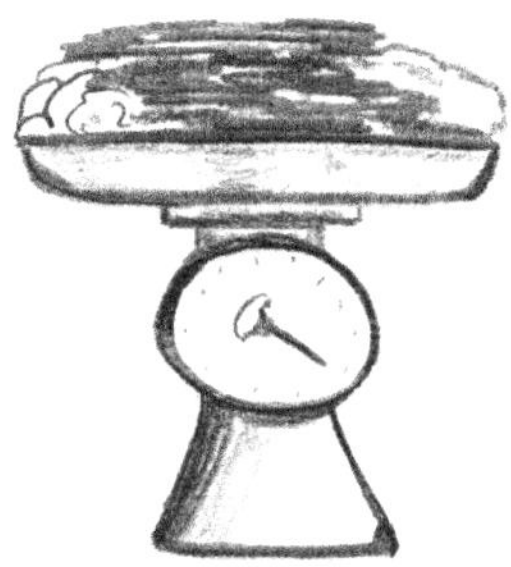

Weighing meat and salt.

7. Use plain salt (even coarse salt) with no added ingredient.

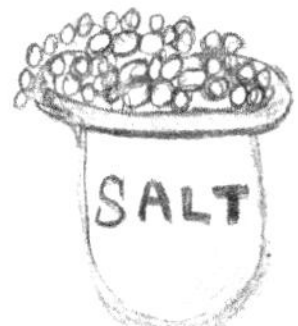

Plain, coarse salt.

8. Use 1 part salt to 3 parts meat.

9. Meat must be cut in less than 2.5 centimeters (1 inch or less) thick strips.

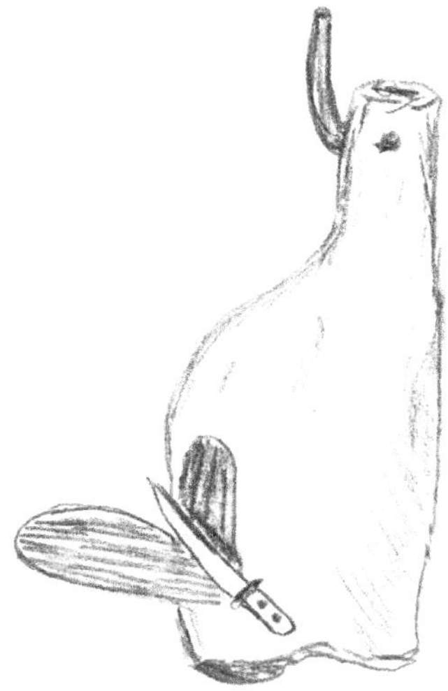

Cutting meat into thin slices.

10. Red meat that is being salted will produce a brine in a day or two.

11. Place a 1.25 centimeters (one-half inch) layer of salt over the bottom of the container.

12. Place a layer of meat completely over the layer of salt.

13. Place the meat strips as close together as possible without overlapping.

14. Cover each layer of meat completely with salt.

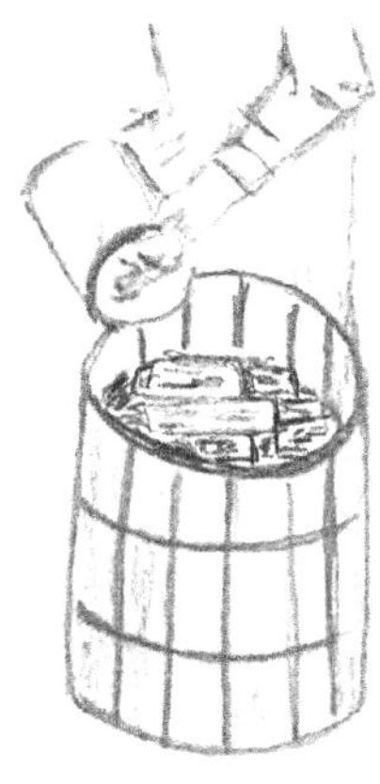

Pouring salt over meat layer.

15. Use plenty of salt over the layer of meat.

16. Continue layering the meat then layering the salt until the container is almost full.

17. The last layer should be salt.

18. Place a clean rock or brick over a piece of clean fabric or burlap to weigh down the brine solution.

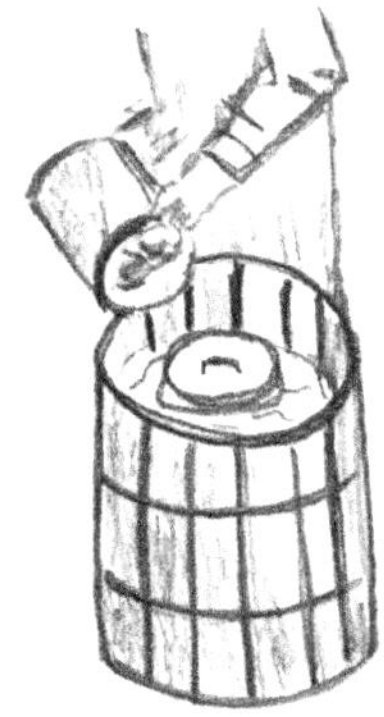

Weight on top of meat in a barrel.

19. The brine (liquid from the muscles) will be produced in a few days and the liquid will cause the meat to float.

20. The meat must be kept below the brine level to cure.

21. If the meat rises above the brine it will spoil and will spoil the entire cure of meat.

22. Meat must be kept in the cure for at least 28 days.

23. The meat must be drained and re-salted several times during the 28 days.

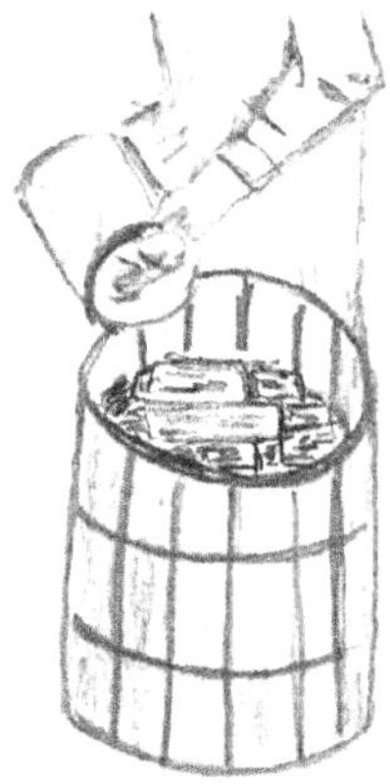

Draining and re-salting meat.

24. After the 28 days, drain the brine and repack with fresh salt.

25. This must be repeated until the meat no longer produces a liquid (brine).

26. The brine solution should never turn sour, thick or ropy.

27. If it does, the brine and meat must be thrown away and the container and the weight cleaned with boiling water.

28. Before eating a salted meat, the meat must be removed from the brine mixture.

29. The meat should be removed from the brine several hours before time to be eaten.

30 The salted meat should be soaked in cold water for several hours.

31. The meat should not be cooked in this solution.

32. The cold water should be emptied and refilled several times.
33. Salty meat may also be boiled to remove the saltiness.
34. This may have to be repeated one or two times.
35. Salted meat should be cooked immediately when removed from the brine.
36. Salted meat may be used in further processed meals, such as stew or soups.
37. Meat that is ground or in small pieces cannot be salted.

Chapter 13
Preservation by Cooling and Freezing

Preservation by Cooling and Freezing

I THESSALONIANS 5:9-11

For God has not appointed us to incur His wrath, but obtain His salvation through our Lord Jesus Christ (the Messiah). Who died for us so that whether we are still alive or are dead, we might live together with Him and share His life.

1. Many countries depend upon cooling and freezing to preserve meat. This method allows for meat to be stored for extended times and should be considered if the capabilities are available.

2. When storing meat either by cooling or freezing, it should be properly wrapped to prevent drying out or moisture getting on the meat.

3. After wrapping meat it should be sorted by cuts of meats and kept in moisture proof boxes or wire baskets.

4. The boxes or baskets may be stacked if the refrigerated air is allowed to move around all sides of the box or basket.

5. Carcasses should be immediately chilled after slaughter bringing the body temperature down quickly to prevent microbial growth. The carcasses should not touch each other, but allow air circulation around each one to cool the individual carcass.

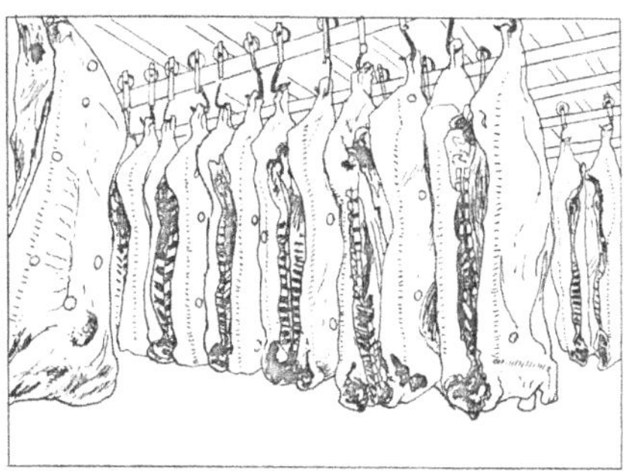

Hot cooler for beef carcasses to chill.
(USDA 1977)

If the carcass will be hot-boned immediately, do not cool it.

Many times it is not possible to cut a carcass up immediately after slaughter. The carcass that is chilled may hang for different lengths of time before it is cut. Do not allow water to splash up on the carcass. Keep the carcass clean and dry.

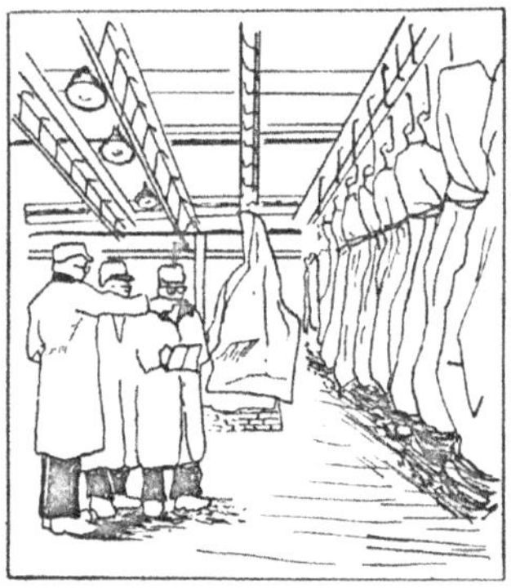

Cooler to hold carcasses. (USDA 1977)

6. Meat cuts and products should be chilled. Refrigeration temperatures are desirable under 9° C (50° F), but the temperature should not freeze 0° C (32° F). If freezing is desired, a unit that is made to freeze should be used.

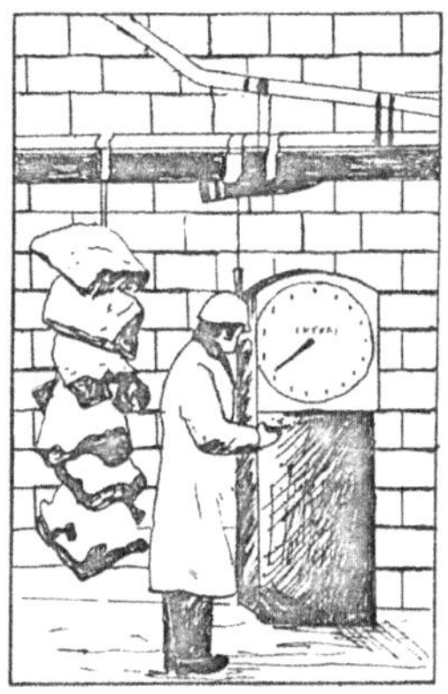

Primal meat cuts being weighed before going into cooler. (USDA 1977)

7. Temperatures in the cooling or freezing unit should remain constant and not be allowed to increase. Freezer temperatures are below freezing and should be maintained until the meat is ready to be prepared and eaten.

8. Refrigeration units come in many sizes and may be constructed with a cooling or freezer unit and a tight closing room, container or case.

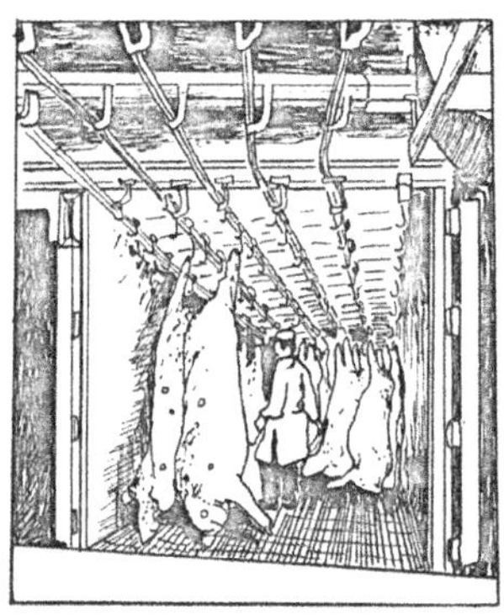

Holding Cooler for Carcasses. (USDA 1977)

9. Coolers may be called Hot Coolers, that store the hot carcasses coming off of the slaughter floor for 24 hours or less and Holding Coolers, that store carcasses for longer periods of time before being further processed or sold.

Suggested Chilling Data from Abattoirs

Body Temperature at Slaughtering	*Final Temperature C (F)*	*Time in coolers (hours)*	*Temperature of coolers C (F)*
Cattle 39 C (102 F)			
Hot Coolers	1 to 1.6 C (34–35 F)	18–24 hours	2.2 to 4.4 C (28–40 F) at 85–90% R.H.
Holding Coolers	1.6 C (35 F)		0 to 1 C (32–34 F) at 90–95% R.H.
Hogs 37.7 to 41 C (100 to 106 F)			
Hot Coolers	2.2 to 3.8 C (36 to 39 F)	16–22 hours	–2.2 to 3.3 C (28 to 38 F)
Hot Cutting			10 C (50 F)
Fresh Pork Holding			–3.3 to –2.2 C (26 to 28 F)
Lambs 36 to 38.8 C (98 to 102 F)			
Hot Coolers	1.1 to 2.2 C (34 to 36 F)	12–14 hours	
Calves			
Hot Coolers	1.1 to 2.2 C (34 to 36 F)	12–18 hours	

Revised from USDA, FSIS Training Manual.

Dressed Weight Ranges of Carcasses being Chilled

Beef	136–454 kg. (300–1,000 lbs.)
Lamb	18–36 kg. (40–80 lbs.)
Hogs	40–205 kg. (90–450 lbs.)
Sheep	28–57 kg. (62–125 lbs.)
Calves	39–159 kg. (85–350 lbs.)

Revised from USDA, FSIS Training Manual.

Chapter 14

Packaging Material for Meat and Meat Products

Packaging Material for Meat and Meat Products

EPHESIANS 5:1-2

Therefore be imitators of God, as well-beloved children imitate their father. And walk in love as Christ loved us and gave Himself up for us, a slain offering and sacrifice to God for you, so that it became a sweet fragrance.

Packaging material requirements

1. Packaging material should be kept in separate rooms that are used exclusively for this purpose and free of dust and vermin.

2. Boxes should be assembled in a sanitary manner, either in a separate room or, if in the processing room, never within 3 meters of exposed product.

3. Packaging material should not be stored on the floor.

4. Waxed assembled boxes should not be nested, unless a liner will be added prior to filling.

5. Assembled boxes with liners should not be nested.

6. Boxes should not be handled by personnel who are handling exposed product.

Pallets in exposed product areas

The use of wooden pallets in areas where there is exposed product should be discontinued if possible. Below are guidelines for using wooden pallets:

1. No wooden pallets should be used within 3 meters of exposed product.

2. All pallets should be clean and structurally sound.

3. Wooden pallets should be covered with a sanitary plastic slip sheet covering the entire top of the pallet.

4. When wooden pallets are used in coolers or freezers, all products present should be hygienically packaged to prevent contact of product with wood.

5. Those establishments which are already using plastic pallets should continue to do so.

Separate storage of packaged and unpackaged products

Unpackaged exposed meat may not be stored in chilling or freezer rooms containing packaged meat. This prevents contamination of the packaging.

Conventional Paper Wrapping

The main purposes of wrapping meat is to prevent contamination and air entering the meat; moisture entering the meat products; and for ease in transportation. These conditions will cause a meat product to have a short storage time.

Meat should be wrapped in wrapping material that will completely cover it and be folded over the sides and ends. There are many wrapping materials available. If none is available even clean newsprint, brown paper or clean fabric would work.

Meat products should be cut in the portions to be used and then wrapped. If a whole carcass is being transported the majority of the carcass should be wrapped to prevent contamination. Meat should be double wrapped if going into the freezer. There are many products available.

Wrapping materials suitable for meats are:

- wax and paraffin-treated kraft papers
- aluminum foil
- laminated foils
- films (polyethylene or polymers)
- food-grade "plastic" dips
- gummy tape for taping ends of paper closed

The characteristics of a good wrapping material include:

- low moisture transmission
- low oxygen permeability
- pliable
- puncture resistant
- non-toxic
- odorless
- easy to mark
- stain proof
- good sealing properties

A good "kraft" paper for meat will have a wax side and a non-wax side that can be written on or an adehesive label attached. If double wrapping, a poly film or foil should be the first layer that will not stick to the meat. The second layer should be a kraft paper.

To wrap meat:

- wrapping should totally enclose the meat
- enclose all ends to prevent moisture entering the package
- "butcher's" wrap is best

The "butcher's" wrap description is below:

The paper should be slightly longer and wider than the piece of meat to be wrapped. The meat should be placed in the center of the paper and the paper ends pulled up to meet and then rolled down tightly downward to meet the meat. This should be a tight fit against the meat. Next, the ends should be pulled tight and each side folded into a triangle and turned under the meat. The second layer of paper should be wrapped as the first layer.

Labeling wrapped meat products

All meat products that have been wrapped should be properly labeled on top of each package in legible, large letters. This may be written directly on the package or on an adhesive label.

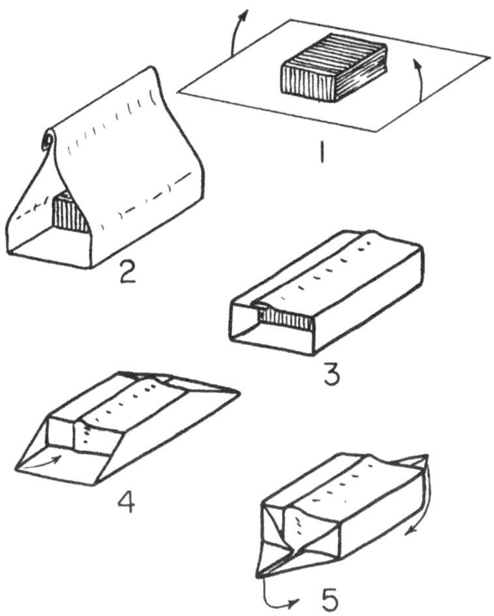

"Butcher" method of wrapping.
(USDA 1978)

The following information should be included on a label:

Date wrapped
Species (beef, lamb, pork, etc.)
Primal or wholesale cut (round, loin, shoulder, etc.)
Subprimal or retail cut (rib steaks, boston roast, etc.)
Owner's name if necessary.

Name of Owner Type of Cut Date Packaged

Label with information.

Vacuum Packaging

There are many types of vacuum packaging equipment. The very basic ones are free standing and can handle up to four smaller pieces of meat. A special vacuum packaging bag is used to place the cut meat inside. The bag is placed inside the vacuum packager. The lid is shut on top of the edge of the bag. The inside air will be "vacuumed" out of the bag and the bag sealed.

This allows sealing of the bag to prevent any air leakage into the bag. The bag may be either refrigerated or frozen for storage.

Cook-in bags (must buy the correct bag) are available. The meat can actually be cooked inside the sealed bag and then eaten or stored for further usage.

The meat color may not be the usual bright red to pinkish color (depends on species) due to the lack of oxygen. Oxygen combines with a meat pigment to give the bright colors associated with fresh meat.

There are more sophisticated and larger pieces of equipment. Different size bags may be purchased for various sizes of meat. The smaller packaging machine can be an asset to the processor.

Advantages of vacuum packing;

1. Removes air to prevent drying out of the meat product
2. Removes air that will allow microorganisms to grow
3. Adds to days that it may be stored under refrigerator conditions
4. Adds to storability in the freezer.

Labels for vacuum packaging may be attached to the outside or added inside the bag.

Name of Owner Type of Cut Date Packaged

Label with information.

Section X

Simple Slaughter and Processing Facility

Chapter 15

Simple Slaughter and Processing Plans and Structure

Simple Slaughter Structure

MATTHEW 7:1-2

Ask, and it shall be given to you; seek, and you shall find; knock, and it shall be opened to you. For everyone who asks receives, and he who seeks finds, and to him who knocks it shall be opened.

The small slaughter facility should involve keeping the *dirty from the clean* parts of the animal. The most important part of a small slaughter facility is to keep it clean. This can be accomplished by slaughtering one animal and then processing it into meat products before slaughtering another animal. A clean up between animals will prevent cross-contamination from one animal to another animal's carcass and meat.

Where available the following items should be included in a structure:

1. Pens to hold animals for slaughter, with water and shade.

2. Concrete floor that slants from back to front. To keep it clean, the concrete floor should extend past the building 3 to 4 meters (10 to 12 feet).

3. A drain with drainage pipe in the center of the concrete floor that drains to the outside and away from the structure.

4. Source of forced water: water pump to a well, pressurized pump with a water reservoir, pressurized pump in a bucket of water, or backpack pressure sprayer with attached tank.

5. Walls at least chest high to prevent pests (vermin) from coming in. Walls should be washable (whitewashed) if available.

6. If at all possible a screening around the structure to prevent pests from coming in.

7. A block and tackle or winch to lift a carcass up off the floor.

8. A bed cradle, if possible, for large animals to lie on while skinning

9. A table for further processing of the animal.

10. Disposal area outside of the facility for internal organs, ingesta and hides until further processed or disposed of.

***Sanitation* is most important in a small slaughter structure.**

1. Before slaughter of the first animal, make sure the inside of the facility is clean and free from litter and vermin.

2. Slaughter one animal at a time, remove the hide and internal parts from the slaughter area and from the inside of the structure. Take the hide and internal parts out to a barrel or other designated area.

3. Rinse down walls, floor and equipment, even between the slaughter of animals.

4. Slaughter one animal, cut the carcass up into smaller portions (process), package and remove the meat products to another facility for storage or sale. This must be done quickly to avoid spoilage of the meat if in hot weather.

5. Totally scrub the walls, concrete floor and equipment with a brush with water and soap and/or Clorox bleach at the end of the last slaughter and processing.

6. Before beginning a new slaughter day, make sure the facility is clean. Rewash walls, floors, table, and equipment if dirty.

7. Keep all wild animals and vermin away from all areas of the facility including the live animals awaiting slaughter. Do not allow these animals to get into the disposed internal parts or hides. Do not allow these animals to eat any scraps from the slaughter facility.

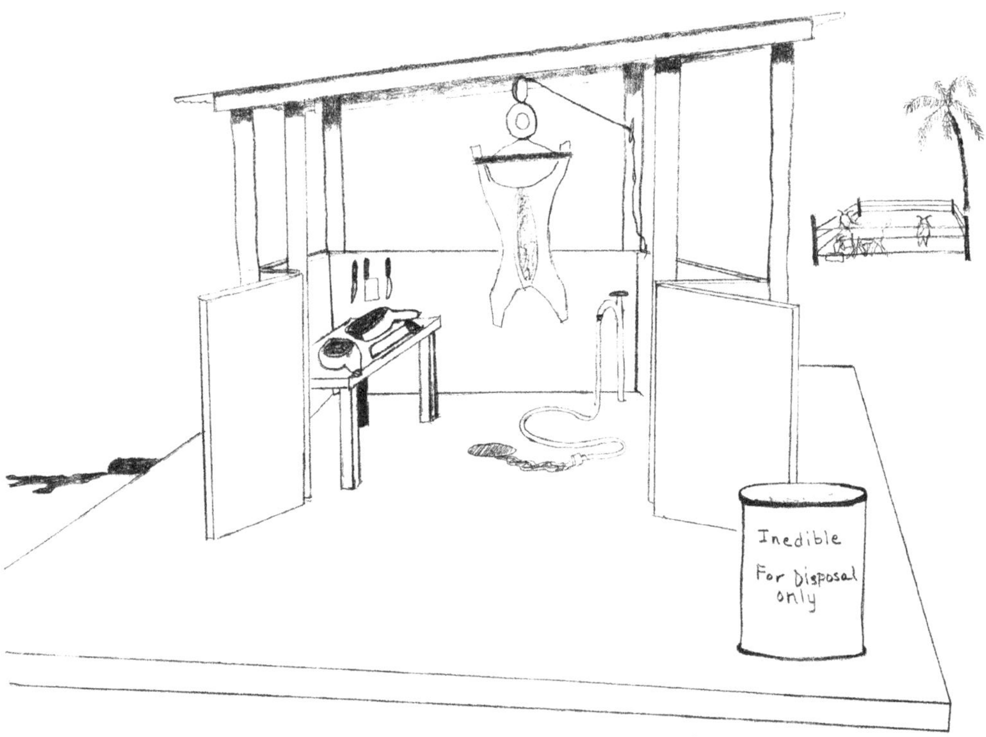

Simple Slaughter and Processing Facility.

Section XI

Small to Medium Sized Slaughter House Plans

Chapter 16

Small Sized Slaughter Facility Plans

Small to Medium Sized Slaughter House Plans

EPHESIANS 1: 4-5

Even as He chose us in Christ before the foundation of the world, that we should be holy and blameless in His sight, even above reproach, before Him in love. For He foreordained us to be adopted as His own children through Jesus Christ, in accordance with the purpose of His will.

This next section of the book is for those who have worked with a simple slaughter and processing structure and would like to increase the size of the facility.

These plans are to give people and communities an idea for potential growth. The plans vary in size and can be used individually or combined to form a larger facility. The plans have no dimensions so the processor can adjust the size according to the number of animals to be slaughtered and processed each day. The plans are divided into Small and Medium Sized Facility. The plans are made to allow for increasing the size depending on the number of animals slaughtered per day.

The locations for the different steps in dressing an animal and sites for inspections are indicated to show a flow in the process. Both plans have an overhead rail system for carcasses placed on trolleys to roll to each process. The overhead rail system can use gravity flow, having a slight downward incline on the rail, to allow the carcass to move freely from the first process to the last. The rail system can also have stops at each process area and the carcasses pushed by workers to each process area along the rail system.

The following factors should determine if an increase is needed:

1. Number of animals slaughtered increases
2. Carcasses are further processed (cut up)
3. Meat is sold to the public in large quantities
4. Improve the sanitation and the inspection standards for the facility
5. Variety of meats offered for sale

There are two plans for the slaughter house:

Plan 1: small slaughter floor (abattoir) only: plan number 1.
Plan 2: medium slaughter floor (abattoir) with attached pens and a boiler room:
Processing Room Plan #1: processing room with separate rooms: storage, freezer, smoke room, kitchen, workers' locker rooms, office, health inspector office, and meat sales room.
Cooler/Chiller: two separate cooler rooms with different number of rails, doors leading from slaughter floor and into process area.

Illustrations of the outside premises are also included of a:

Small Sized Slaughter and Processing Facility
Medium Sized Slaughter and Processing Facility

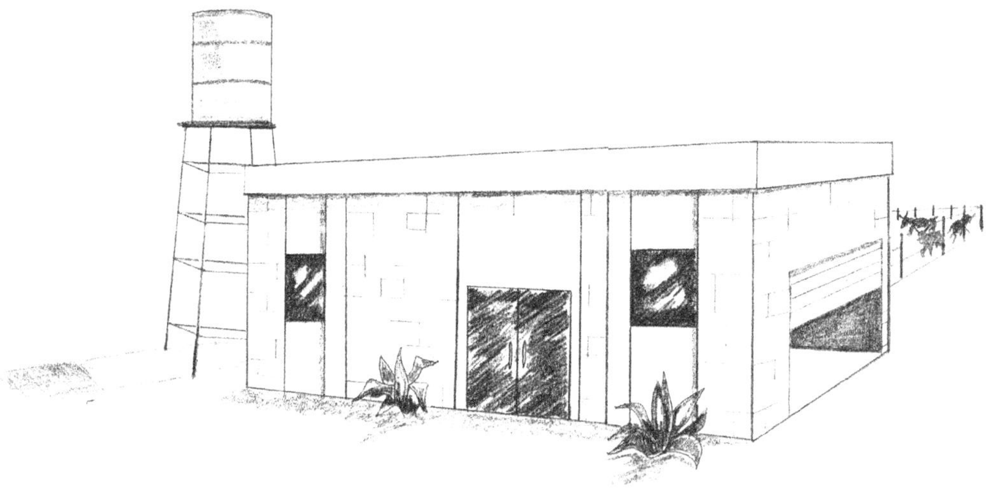

Small Slaughter and Processing Facility.

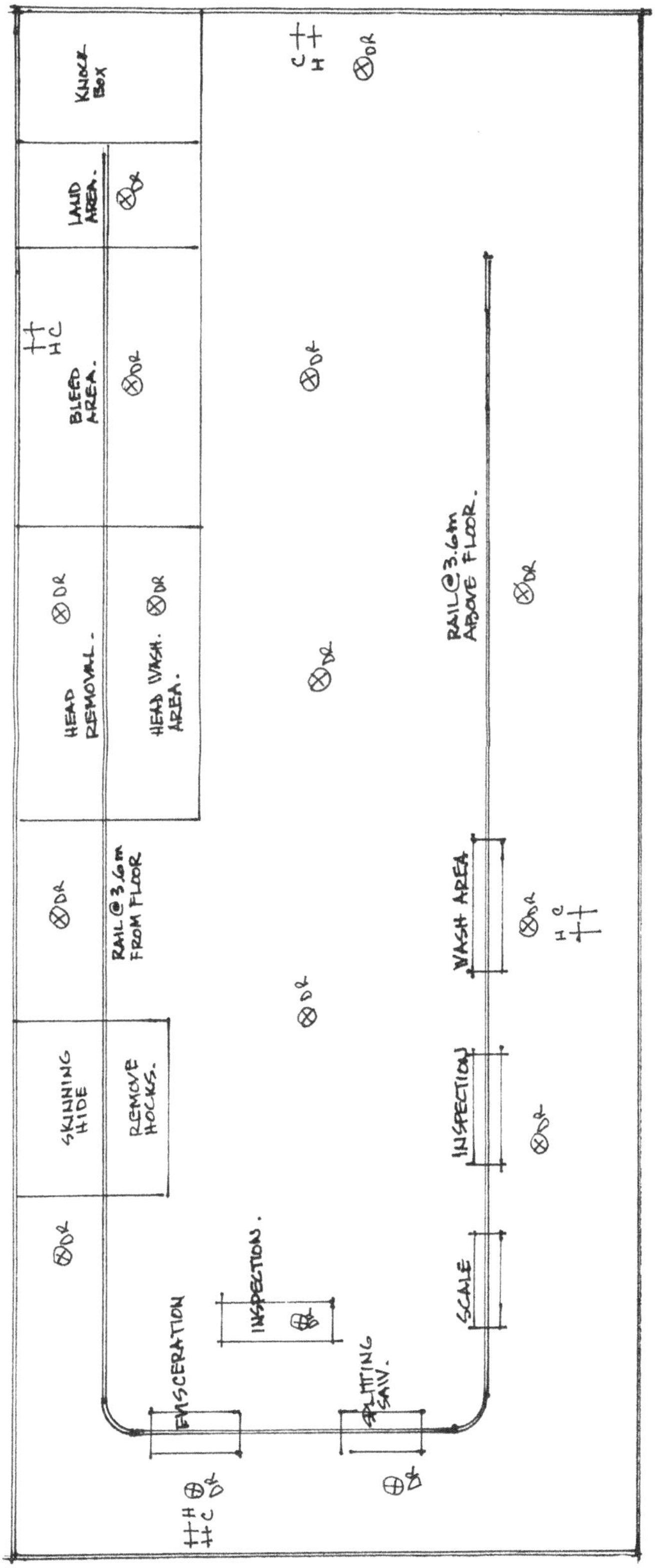

SLAUGHTER FLOOR - PLAN 1

Chapter 17

Medium Sized Slaughter and Processing Facility Plans

II CORINTHIANS 5:21

For our sake He made Christ to be sin Who knew no sin, so that in and through Him we might become the righteousness of God.

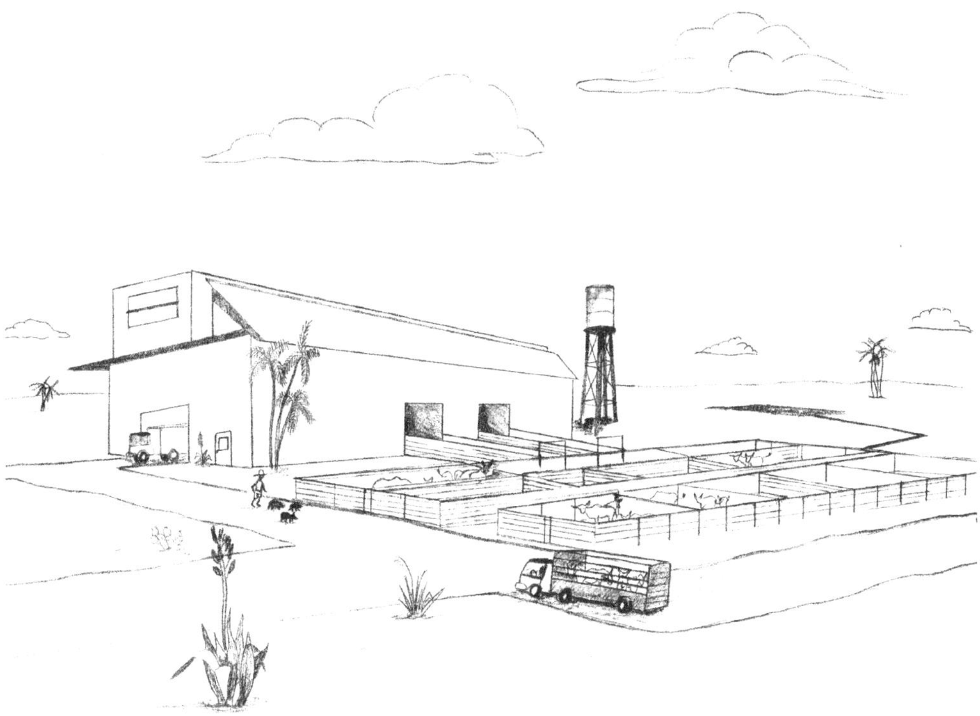

Medium Sized Slaughter and Processing Facility.

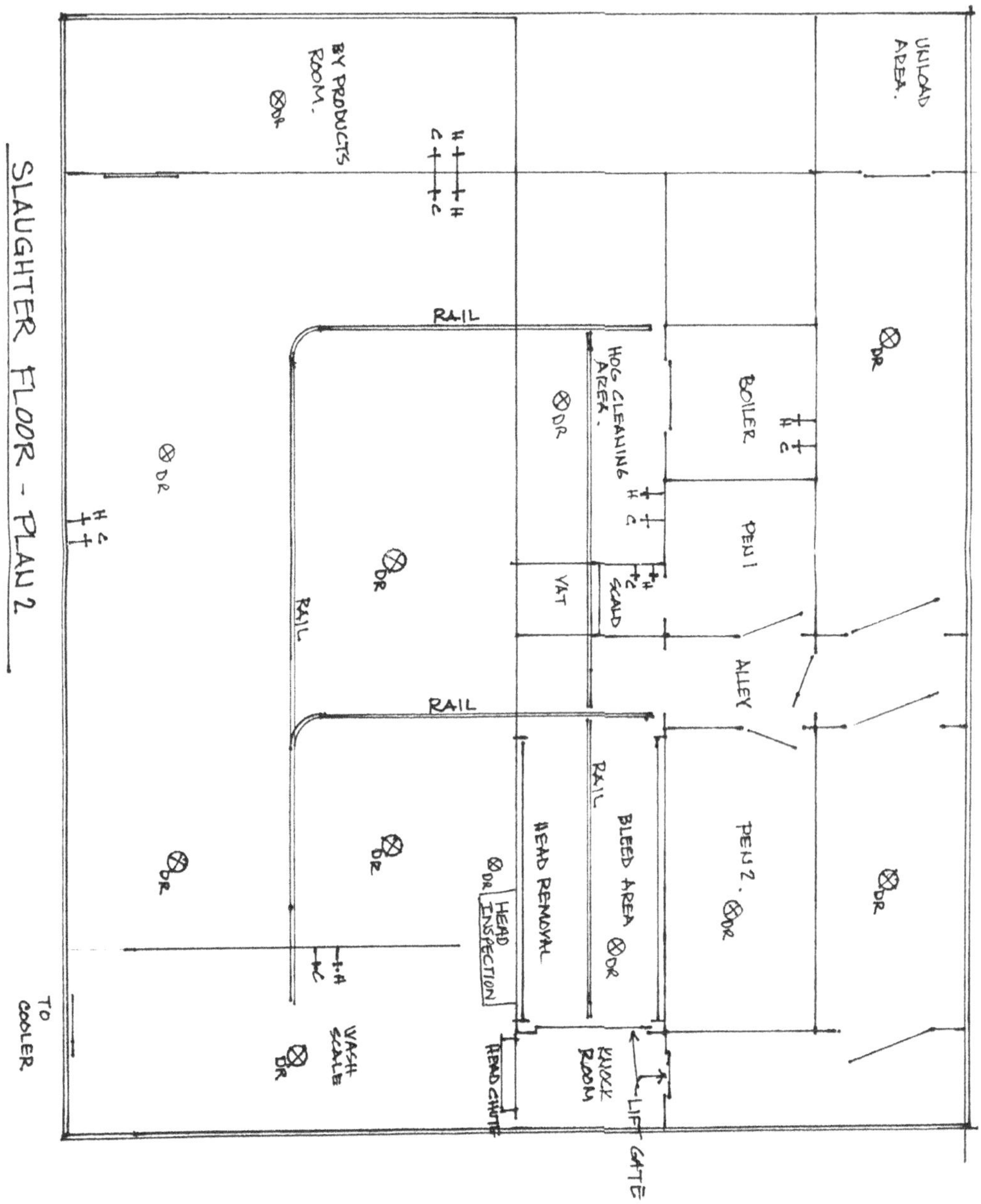
SLAUGHTER FLOOR - PLAN 2
UNLOAD AREA.
BY PRODUCTS ROOM.
RAIL
HOG CLEANING AREA.
BOILER
PEN 1
VAT
SCALD
ALLEY
RAIL
RAIL
BLEED AREA
PEN 2.
HEAD REMOVAL
HEAD INSPECTION
WASH SCALE
KNOCK ROOM
LIFT GATE
HEAD CHUTE
TO COOLER
DR
H
C

Chapter 18

Processing Room Plan

Romans 6:11

Even so consider yourselves also dead to sin and your relation to it broken, but alive to God [living in unbroken fellowship with Him] in Christ Jesus.

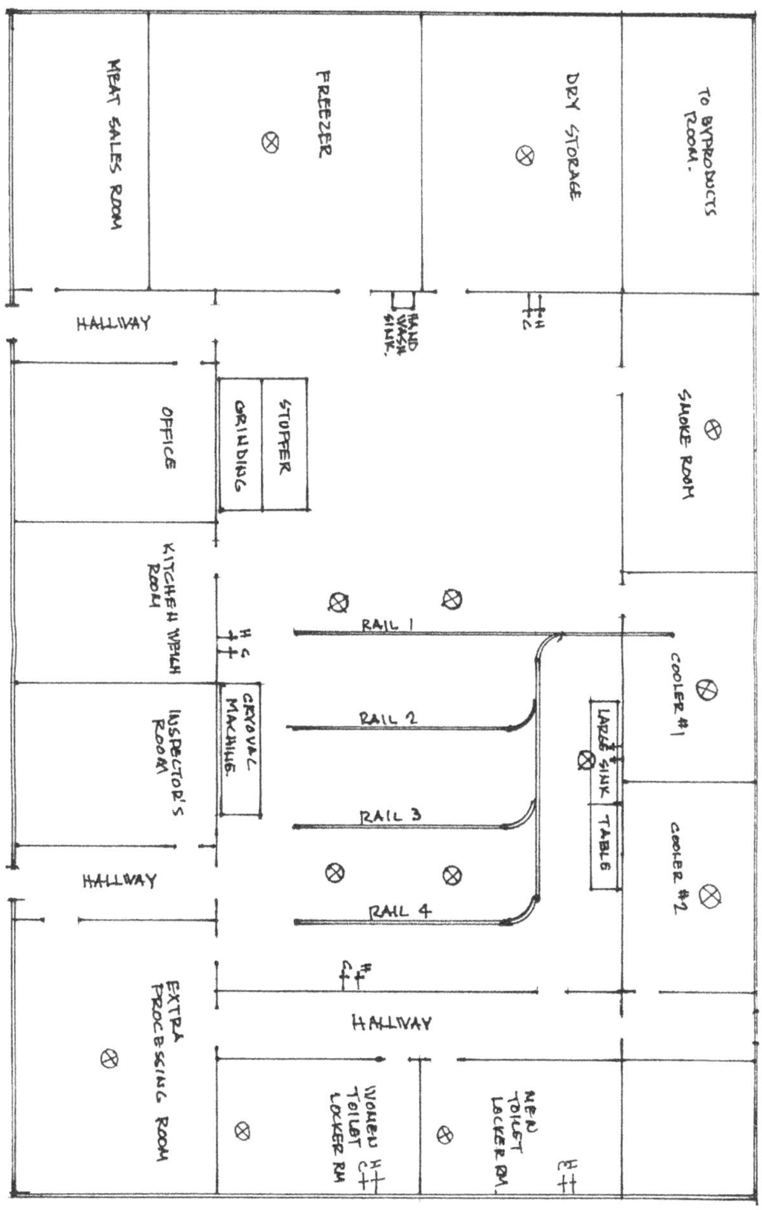

PROCESSING ROOM PLAN #1

Chapter 19
Cooler/Chilling Room Plan

John 5:30

I am able to do nothing from Myself. Even as I hear, I judge and My judgment is right (just, righteous), because I do not seek or consult My own will but only the will and pleasure of the Father Who sent Me.

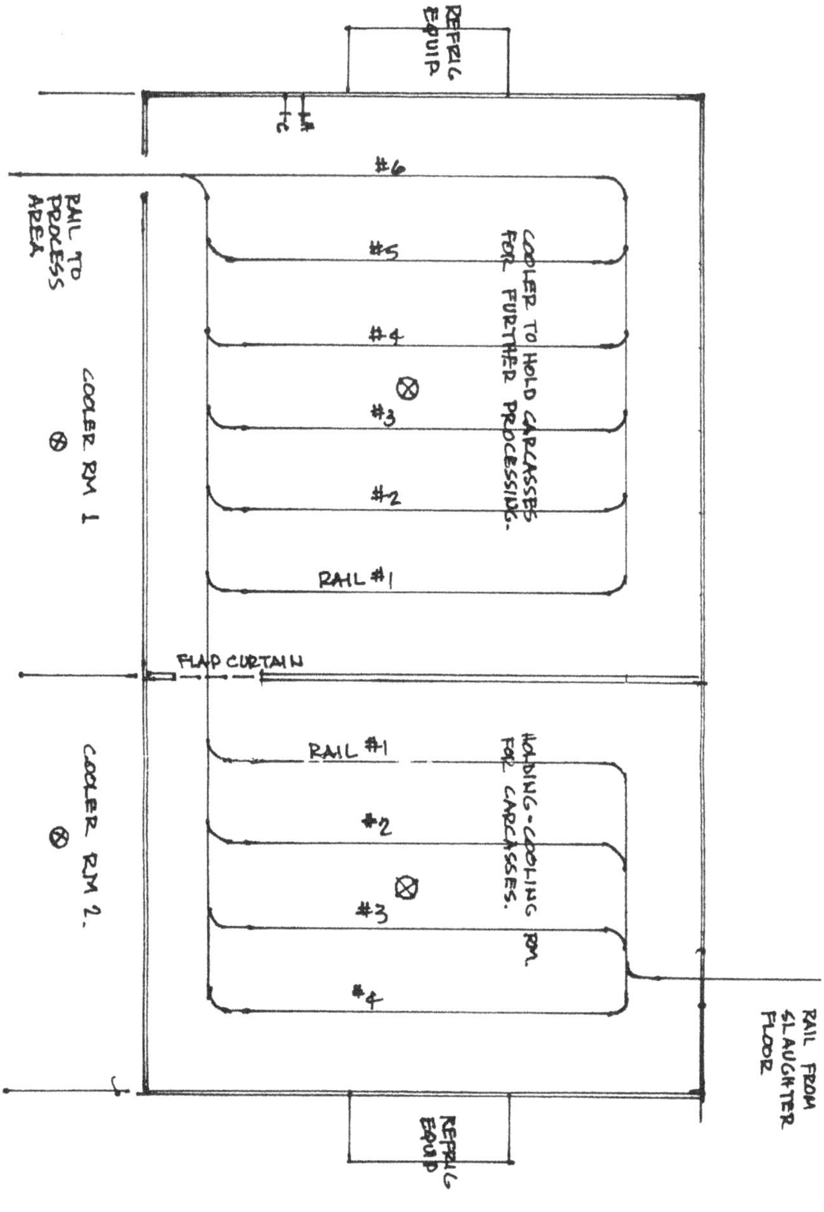

COOLER / CHILLING ROOMS.

Chapter 20

Facilities for Meat Slaughter and Processing Plants—General Guidelines

Facilities for Meat Slaughter and Processing Plants—General Guidelines

Psalm 36:6

Thy righteousness is like the mountains of God; Thy judgments are like a great deep. O Lord, Thou preservest man and beast.

Location:

Location for the facility should be in a sanitary environment.

The facility should be separated from other businesses and have room for buildings and pens.

Size:

The size should include buildings, roads in and out, room for more buildings in the future, and areas for people to park vehicles or walk up to the facility.

The site should be away from any trash areas, landfills or junk areas that may allow vermin (rodents, cats, dogs, lizards, flies, etc.) to live.

The direction of the wind is important. Winds should not carry any other odors or substances for other businesses or industry to the facility. The odors or substances could cause problems with the live animals and the condition of the meat.

Flow of Operations

A good facility should have a flow of operations, so that the animals and meat products all flow are in one direction and do not cross each other. This prevents cross contamination and possible future problems.

The flow should begin with the live animal, then go into the slaughter facility. The slaughter area should never go back across the area where live animals are brought in or housed.

Trash containers should be out of the way of food products, so not to contaminate the food products.

Rooms need to be large enough to contain the equipment and supplies needed for the slaughter or processing steps.

People can carry many contaminants onto a slaughter floor or processing floor. It is necessary to have a flow of traffic, so people are not walking in and moving across areas that they may contaminate.

People working with live animals should not be in processing areas. People working in processing areas should not be in the area of live animals.

Toilets and areas for people to change clothes should be away from slaughter and processing areas.

Separation of Raw and Cooked Products

Raw products may contaminate cooked products. If there are any cooked products they should be in a separate area from raw meat products.

Cooked product areas should be separate from other areas of the facility including raw meat product cutting rooms, carcass coolers and slaughter floors.

The area for cooked products should have little movement of people to prevent contamination.

Cooked product needs to be covered and stored in proper facilities: coolers or freezers.

Dry storage, packing material, locker rooms, and rooms to make up boxes should be near cooked products room, but not in the same room as the cooked meat products.

Perishable Product

Meat products that can spoil easily by microorganism growth should be kept in a separate room from any products that may contaminate them.

Edible and Inedible Products

Edible products are meat and meat products that are for human food. Edible products may become contaminated from sewage, stomach contents, hides, condemned animal parts and organs.

Edible products should be kept in a separate room and storage from inedible. Inedible products are meat and meat products that are not for human food because of disease or contamination.

People working in the inedible product area should not go into the edible product area or room. Edible product workers should not go into the inedible product area or room to prevent cross-contamination.

Inedible product area or room should be clearly marked and separate from the edible meat product area. Equipment used in edible meat products should not be near the inedible product area or room.

Inedible products may be further processed for use for animal food. The inedible products may be denatured, cooked or rendered in a way so that it will not go into human food. The area or room for inedible products should be large enough for this process to occur. The area or room should be large enough for packing and even storing the inedible product until it can be moved from the facility.

Dry Storage

Dry storage is an area or room where products that must be kept dry and clean are stored. The products in this area may include wrapping paper, boxes, tape, clothing, spices, and other products.

If possible, it is good to have shelves or pallets to place the dry storage product on to prevent it from becoming dirty and contaminated from sitting on the floor. Shelves keep the product dry by keeping it up off the floor, if there should be water leakage into the area or room.

Coolers and Freezers

Coolers and freezers should have space to store product. Shelves or pallets will keep the product up off the floor and separate. Coolers and freezers should be made out of material that can be cleaned, is resistant to water and moisture, and non-corrosive.

A freezer door should be made from a material that will not easily freeze and should be moisture resistant.

Employee Facilities

Employee facilities should be separate from all areas of operation and in a location that the employees do not have to walk through a processing, dry storage, cooler, or slaughter area to reach.

The locker room should be clean and designed to prevent cross contamination of meat products. The dressing area should be separate from the toilet area and should provide privacy. If a shower is available it should also provide privacy, be separate from the toilet area, and be kept clean with fresh running water.

Lockers, if available, should be separate from all processing, dry storage, cooler, or slaughter areas. The lockers should be large enough for the workers to store clothes and other items. The lockers should be made of a material that can be easily cleaned and is non-corrosive.

Drinking water for employees should come from a clean water supply used for human consumption (potable water). It should be allowed to drain directly into a drainage system and not run into a processing, dry storage, cooler, or slaughter area.

Hand wash sinks

Hand wash sinks or hand wash area with potable running water and soap should be provided for the workers to wash their hands after using the toilet or the locker room. This will prevent cross contamination from the workers to the meat products.

Hand wash sinks should have both hot and cold water, soap, disposable towels, and a trash can. A hand wash sink should be close to each work area and also the inspector's inspection area.

Construction

The building for slaughter should be constructed of a material that can be cleaned. The material should be durable, with non-toxic and non-corrosive materials. The material should not allow moisture to go into it. A light color with a surface that is easy to clean should be considered.

Wood should not be used if possible. If wood is used, it should be smooth and sealed with a sealant that will prevent moisture from going into the wood. Also, this sealant will prevent the wood from splintering and going into meat products. Wood should not be painted because it will peel.

Floors

Floors should be made of a material that is easily cleaned. Floors may be made of tile, cut stone, or concrete. The floor should have a rough surface to prevent workers from slipping on the material.

A slope to the floor will allow water to run off and prevent standing water.

If a curb is used around a floor to indicate separation of areas, the curbs should be high up the walls and also made of a material that is easily cleaned.

Interior Walls

The finished surface of the walls should also be made of a material that will be easily cleaned and will not stain. The walls should also be of a material that will not contaminate carcasses and meat products if they should touch it.

Walls should be smooth and any seams between sections of the wall should be sealed off to prevent moisture from seeping into the wall.

Ceilings and Overhead Structures.

Ceilings and overhead structures should be made of material that does not need to be painted or plastered. The ceiling should not be of a material that will allow water to accumulate and drip onto the meat products.

The ceiling should be easily cleaned and not have anything that can drop from the ceiling to contaminate the carcasses or meat products. Concrete is a good material for ceilings.

Windows

Windows may contaminate meat products. Dirt, vermin, water and even broken glass can be contaminates. A protection (screen) should be over outside windows to prevent vermin, birds, lizards and insects from coming into the facility. Window ledges should have a slope to prevent dirt and debri from accumulating on the ledge.

The window sill needs to be up off the floor to prevent damage to the window from workers and equipment. Window panes should be made of shatter proof material such as a type of plastic.

Doors

Doors should not be a source of contamination. The door should be made of a material that is easily cleaned and will keep insects, vermin, other contaminants and material out of the room or area. The door should be made of a material that will not allow moisture to go into it. The door should be tight fitting to prevent air, insects and vermin from moving into the room or area that it opens into.

Doors should be wide and high enough to allow material to move through the door without touching the door. The door should be durable.

There are many types of doors that are used for specific areas of production.

Ventilation

Ventilation should be in all areas of the facility. Air can contaminate with insects, dust, odors or water vapors. Ventilation will allow this air to be removed from the processing area. Screens and filters should be used to prevent outside contaminants from coming into the facility.

Lighting

Light is important to the sanitation of the slaughter and processing facility. It is important for the safety of the workers, but also for inspection of animals, carcasses, and meat products to be completed. Light fixtures in the facility should be of a material or a cover that will not break. The light fixtures should be able to withstand water and prevent dirt and debris from attaching to the light fixtures.

A foot candle is the measurement of lighting. Minimum lighting intensity should be between 30 foot candles to 50 foot candles. The higher foot candles are needed in inspection areas of live animals, carcasses and meat products.

Poultry facilities require up to 200 foot candles for inspection areas.

Guidelines for Minimum Lighting Intensity in Meat Establishments

Area	*30 ft. candles*	*50 ft. candles*
General lighting (area where animals are killed, eviscerated, and products are processed or packaged)	X	
Offal cooler	X	
Carcass coolers	X	
Freezers	X	
Dry storage	X	
Ante-mortem inspection	X	
Suspect pen inspection area		X
Inspection stations		X
Establishment quality control inspection areas		X
Recondition and re-inspection areas		X
All other areas	X	

Guidelines for Minimum Lighting Intensity in Poultry Establishments

Area	*30 ft. candles*	*50 ft. candles*	*200 ft. candles*
Ante-mortem inspection	X		
Inspection station (traditional)		X	
Inspection station (NELS/SIS/NTI)			X
Pre and post chill inspection areas			X
Reconditioning and re-inspection areas			X
Establishment quality control inspection areas			X
All other areas	X		

Water Supply

Water should be fresh, clean and have pressure. The water that is used for slaughter and meat processing is potable water. Potable water is safe for human food products. The water supply should be inspected by an agency or service.

Cross contamination of spent or used water with fresh, clean water should be avoided. This could happen with back flow or a siphonage that goes back to the fresh water. The pipes that carry the clean water should be clearly marked and installed in a way that it will not cross with non-potable (not for human consumption) water.

Care should be given to have the plumbing checked by a health professional or inspector. Water used around live animals and on the slaughter floor should be drained to a separate area away from the water supply. The water supply from coolers, boilers, cleaning systems should also have a separate drain system.

Drains and Seals

A good facility will have floor drains that come to one point (area) that can then be drained away. A point or area drain collects water from a specific area. The floor should be sloped to allow the water to drain into that point drain.

A trench drain is another drain that collects water from a larger area and then directs it to a larger drain. The floor should be sloped towards the trench drain. Drains should flow away from the product direction of flow. The drains should be located in areas that are easily cleaned and out of the main flow of traffic.

Trap seals are found within floor drains. The trap seals have vents that direct air from the drains toward the outside. Trap seals prevent sewage odors from moving into the facility.

Drainage Lines and Cleanouts

Drainage lines must be set with local health requirements. The lines should be leak proof and have rodent screens or traps to prevent vermin from moving up the lines into the facility. Covers could be used to prevent debris from blocking the lines and also to keep out vermin.

A cleanout should be in the drainage system to prevent the sewer from blocking. Cleanouts should be easily reached and located in areas where it would not contaminate the meat products.

Sewage

A sewage system should be designed to comply with the local code requirements. If there are no code requirements, the sewage system should be designed as not to contaminate the ground and water supply.

Sewage may carry microorganisms that can cause humans to become ill. Sewage should not come in contact with any meat products, equipment, or any areas where meat is being prepared.

The sewage system should be large enough to handle the amount of sewage that is produced daily by the facility. The system should be built so that it can be enlarged. The sewage system should be away from the product, ingredient and packaging areas.

Rewritten from Federal Register, Vol. 62., No. 164., Monday, August 24, 1997. Rules and Regulations. USDA/NCDA & CS Facility Guidelines for Meat Processing Plants.

Chapter 21

Meat Slaughter General Facility Guidelines

Meat Slaughter General Facility Guidelines

Revelation 21:4

God will wipe away every tear from their eyes; and death shall be no more, neither shall there be anguish nor grief nor pain any more, for the old conditions and the former order of things have passed away.

Livestock Pens

Pens should be designed in a way to prevent contamination of the hides of the animals that would contaminate the carcasses in the slaughter. The pens should be designed to prevent any injury to the animals. There should not be any sharp objects that could injure the animals in movement to and from the pens and inside the pens. This also is important with any walkways and openings into and out of the pens.

The livestock pen should be located outside of the slaughter area to prevent contaminates of dust, mud, and other debri. The pens should have water troughs for the animals. Pens should be placed in an area where there will be no standing water or muddy areas from water troughs.

The floor of the pen, walkways, and ramps should provide good footing for the animals. A material that will not injure the animals, yet be easy to clean should be used. Floors should be at a slope for easy cleaning. If possible, a water source with hose connections should be close by for cleaning the pens.

Pens should be sturdy and high enough so livestock cannot escape or injure themselves. All fences, gates, and chutes should be made of a material that is easily cleaned. The pens should have a small gate that will allow a man to move through to prevent injury to himself. If there is only a wall, there should be a way made for the people to be able to climb the wall quickly.

The pens should be in an area where the animal health inspector can move around and look at the animals before slaughter. The pens should be large enough for the animals to be comfortable and able to lie down and move around. The pen should be large enough for the animals to be moved so all sides can be observed by the inspector.

A covered pen should be made for injured or crippled animals. The pen should be large enough to allow the animal to get up and move around. There should be an area for water and food within reach of the animal.

A suspect (sick) pen should be available and separate from the other livestock pens. This pen is designed for the animal health inspector to be able to examine the animal. The suspect pen should have drainage away from the other livestock pens to prevent any disease from reaching healthy animals.

Slaughter Area

The slaughter area should be kept separate from the outside by a wall or fence that can withstand moisture and is easily cleaned. The wall should have a door that will close on its own to prevent insects and vermin from entering the slaughter area. The slaughter area is difficult to keep sanitary, so attention should be given to keep it as clean as possible during the slaughter operations.

Slaughter area should be continually moving a clean product away from the area where live animals are brought in. Once an animal is stunned and bled it will be moving from an unsanitary condition towards a sanitary condition as a carcass. Once the hide is removed it should be taken from the slaughter area and not moved through the area of a hanging or hideless carcass. The hide should be kept on the unsanitary side of the slaughter area.

The offal or the insides of the animal should also not be moved under the hideless or dressed carcass to prevent contamination. The offal should be moved into an area away from the carcasses for further cleaning.

The workers should not walk through the dressed carcasses moving into and out of the slaughter area. This will reduce contamination on the carcasses. The slaughter area floor space should allow sanitary slaughter operations and allow room for inspection.

Stunning Areas

Stunning areas should have flooring that will prevent the animal from slipping. Chutes or holding pens should be large enough for the size of animal. There should be no sharp objects, boards, nails, exposed equipment in the pathway to the stunning area or in the stunning area that might injure the animal or the workers. The floor should not have holes that the animal could step in and lose its footing or injure itself. The area should be kept clean and dry to prevent contamination of the hide.

If a captive bolt stunner is being used, the holding pen or chute should hold the animal tight enough for the worker to stun the animal correctly. Shackles should be easily accessible to hoist the animal up, if it will be hoisted immediately after stunning or in ritualistic slaughter.

If electrical stunning is used, the stunning area should be constructed so that any electrical devices will not cause injury to the animal before it is stunned.

Rail Arrangement

Rails should be arranged to provide enough room for carcasses to move without touching equipment, walls, structural columns, parts of the building or other carcasses to prevent contamination.

Rail arrangement will be determined with the type of rail and the speed of carcasses moving down the rail.

Trim rails should be the last rail before the final carcass inspection area.

Carcasses should not be contaminated by water and debris splashing up from the floor in the cooler/storage area. The clearance from the lowest point of the carcass to the highest point of the floor, should be considered with the rail height in the cooler.

Viscera Separation and Edible Byproducts

Viscera and edible byproducts (organs and offal) are cleaned and separated in areas where microorganism would easily grow. The facility area for separation of the viscera should have a designated pan or truck to handle the viscera. The viscera between various species should not be mixed (co-mingled).

It is very important to avoid the cross contamination of viscera and byproducts with other meat products. A separate cooler should be provided to hold the edible organs and offal under refrigeration.

This area or cooler should be easily reached by the workers. The workers must not cross through a line of carcasses or a cooler full of carcasses to reach this area. This will prevent cross contamination from the organs and offal and the carcasses.

Carcass Washing

Washing carcasses after inspection is important to remove any bone dust or other contamination. The wash area should be separate from the incoming animals and carcass with hide on. The wash area should have a sloping floor with an adequate drain. The wash area if possible should have a platform for the worker to stand on to wash all parts of the carcass.

Retain Room/Area

Carcasses that have a disease or abnormality that should be further inspected by a trained inspector should be isolated from the rest of the carcasses. All of the organs, offal, and head, in question should remain with the carcass. The area to keep this carcass should be marked "Retained".

If the carcass is to be retained in the cooler, an area with mesh wire that is water resistant may be constructed to surround the carcass and also have a gate that can be locked.

Rewritten from Federal Register, Vol. 62., No. 164., Monday, August 24, 1997. Rules and Regulations. USDA/NCDA & CS Facility Guidelines for Meat Processing Plants

Chapter 22
Additional Guidelines for Different Species

Additional Guidelines for Different Species

LUKE 12:24

Observe and consider the ravens; for they neither sow nor reap, they have neither storehouse nor barn; and yet God feeds them. Of how much more worth are you than the birds!

Cattle Slaughter

Cattle facilities can be of many different types depending on the number of animals slaughtered, and the rate and type of inspection.

Rail Heights, Distances, and other cattle slaughter area dimensions

Guidelines for Distances in Cattle Slaughtering Establishments

Area/Activity	*Vertical Distance*	*Horizontal Distance*
Bleeding rail (distance from rail to point of application of shackle to shackle foot—1.2 m (4 ft.)	4.9 m (16 feet)	
Dressing rails (trolley length—0.4 m (1 ft 3 in)	3.7 m (12 feet 3 inches)	
Beef cooler rails (trolley length—0.4 m (1 foot 3 inches)	3.4 m (11 feet)	
Moving equipment—heights of conveyor rails, platforms, top of viscera inspection table		
Dry landing area in front of stunning pen.		2.1 by 2.5 m (7 by 8 feet)
Curb of bleeding area to pitch plates (no header rails)		1.5 m (5 feet)
Between header rail and carcass washing rail, if parallel		1.8 m (6 feet)
Between header or washing rails and wall of slaughtering room		0.9m (3 feet)
Between center lines of dressing beds		2.5 m (8 feet)
Between moving top table and dressing rail at inspector's platform		1.7 m (5 feet 6 inches)
Area for sterilizing viscera inspection truck		2.1 by 2.5 m (7 by 8 feet)

When rails are involved in horizontal distance measurements, the distance is measured from the center of the rail. When rails are involved in vertical distance measurements, the distance is measured from the top of the rail to the highest part of the floor.

Dry Landing Area

A dry landing area should be adjacent to the stunning pen or area. This landing area should be large enough for the livestock. The dry landing area should be located and drained separate from the bleeding area. The dry landing area should be enclosed with a high and sturdy fence to prevent the escape of an animal that has not be adequately stunned.

Bleeding Area

A curbed bleeding area or a container to collect the blood from the animal being bled will prevent it from contaminating carcasses nearby. The bleeding area should be located so that the blood will not be splashed into the stunning area, dry landing area, or skinning area.

A curb around the bleeding area is good to keep the blood in the area. A floor drain used to collect blood should slope downward to allow blood to flow away from the bleeding area. A water outlet with a hose connection should be nearby to hose down the area after each animal is bled.

Head Removal Area

Head removal areas need to be away from carcasses and the rumen contents. There should be space to dehorn, wash and inspect heads. There should be room to store heads and an area for head workup away from carcass contamination. A head wash cabinet provides this protection and an area to clean up the heads for further processing.

Hide Removal

Once hides are removed from a carcass they should be moved to an area away from the carcasses to prevent contamination. A separate area or room for storage and working hides should be provided away from any carcass and meat product processing. The area should have a drain and a hose connection to clean up after hides have been removed. The area should be ventilated to allow airborne contaminates to be removed from the area.

Feet and Udders

Once feet and udders are removed from the carcass they should be placed in a separate area or holding container to prevent splashing of milk on the carcass and further contamination from the feet.

Working Areas

If carcasses are hung on a rail, the carcasses should be high enough on the rail to prevent them from dragging across workers feet and bodies or the platforms on which they may be standing.

Viscera Trucks

A viscera truck in smaller facilities is easy to manage and to help move the offal and edible organs away from the carcass. The viscera truck also gives the inspector an area in which to examine the viscera. The viscera truck should be made of a material that can be easily washed and sterilized. The washing area for the viscera truck should be away from carcasses and edible meat products.

Post-mortem Inspection Station and Retain Rail

An inspection station after the final trim should be made up of 1.5 m (5 feet) of unobstructed line space for each inspector. This gives the inspector adequate room to inspect the carcass or head.

A minimum of 50 foot candles without shadows should be available at the head, viscera, and carcass inspection areas.

For inspectors of viscera and head on cattle, a sterilizer should be located adjacent to the inspector's work area. A hand wash sink with hot and cold water, soap, disposable towels, and trash can should also be adjacent to the inspector's work area.

Calf, Sheep, and Goat Slaughter

Guidelines for Distances in Calf, Sheep, and Goat Slaughtering Facilities

Item	*Vertical Distance*	*Horizontal Distance*
Bleeding rail for calves (distance from top of rail to point of application of shackle to shackled foot (0.8 m)—2 feet 6 inches	3.3 m (11 feet)	
Bleeding rails if only sheep or goats are slaughtered	2.7 m—3.4 m (9 feet—11 feet)	
Dressing rail (trolley length 0.3 m (1 foot)	2.6 m (8 feet 6 inches)	
Cooler rails, calf carcasses 0.3 m (1 foot)	2.6 m (8 feet 6 inches)	
Moving equipment		
Vertical of rail to edge of viscera inspection stand		0.6 m (2 feet)
Length of rail from point of evisceration to point where carcass inspection is completed		1.8 m (6 feet)

When rails are involved in horizontal distance measurements, the distance is measured from the center of the rail. When rails are involved in vertical distance measurements, the distance is measured from the top of the rail to the highest part of the floor.

Hog Slaughter

When building or modifying a facility for slaughtering hogs these additional guidelines should be considered.

Livestock pens

Hogs can easily overheat; the holding pen should have a roof and a water system to shower the hogs when temperatures are greater than 21° C (70° F).

Operations Areas

To prevent contamination the following operations should be located in an area separate from the carcass final dressing area to prevent contamination:

hoisting, sticking, and bleeding
scalding vat
dehairing machine within a curbed area with a drainage outlet that will not clog
gabrelling table
singeing operation

Rail Arrangements for Hogs

Guidelines for Distances in Hog Slaughtering Facilities

Item	*Vertical distance*
Bleeding rail to sticker's area	3.2 m (10 feet 6 inches)
Extension of bleeding rail to top of scalding vat	2.7 m (9 feet)
Dressing rails	3.3 m (11 feet)
Gambrels (suspending carcasses to floor) ((0.3 m) (1 foot))	3 m (10 feet)
Distances from rail to bottom of inspection pans and various foot platforms	
Rails in coolers for hog carcasses with heads removed ((0.3 m) (1 foot))	2.7 m (9 feet)
Rails to coolers for carcasses with heads attached ((3m) (1 foot))	3 m (10 feet)
Vertical of dressing rail to various foot platforms and widths of platforms	

When rails are involved in vertical distance measurements, the distance is measured from the top of the rail to the highest part of the floor.

Scalding

To avoid contamination of the carcass, a scalding tank or barrel is used to remove hair and other contaminants on the animal.

Shaving, singeing, and carcass washing

A shaving rail should be available for hogs that need more hair removed before head dropping. If on a moving chain, a singer should have an easy off/on switch to prevent hogs from burning.

Inspection

On a moving line, the areas for post-mortem inspection should be 1.5 m (5 feet) of line space for each head or carcass inspector.

A minimum of 50 foot candles of shadowless lighting at the inspection area for the head, viscera, and carcass should be provided.

A hand wash sink with soap, disposable towels, hot and cold water, and trash can should be adjacent to the inspector's work area

A sterilizer should be at each inspection area on the line.

Rewritten from Federal Register, Vol. 62., No. 164., Monday, August 24, 1997. Rules and Regulations. USDA/NCDA & CS Facility Guidelines for Meat Processing Plants

Section XII

Further Processing of Carcasses

Processing of Animal Carcasses

This section describes in detail how to further process a beef, pork, and lamb (small ruminant) carcass into primal and retail cuts that are utilized in the larger countries such as the United States and Canada. Retail cuts popular in these countries include individual sized cuts of meat, ground meat, and roasts that can be slowly cooked. This may give people other ways to market the meat.

Carcasses are traditionally cut in the manners described and for the following reasons:

Cuts:
1. Cut bony from less bony meat cuts.
2. Cut leaner (less fat) meat cuts from fatter (less lean) meat cuts.
3. Cut thinner meat cuts from thicker meat cuts.
4. Cut more tender cuts of meat from tougher cuts of meat.

Reasons:
1. More individual cuts of meat
2. Easier storage
3. Easier transport

Cleanliness of Facility

The facility should be clean before cutting the carcass. After each carcass is cut, clean the equipment and tables, then begin to cut a new carcass. Pork can carry parasites than can transfer to beef and lamb. It is advised to cut beef and lamb separate from pork. The pork may even be cut last, then the area cleaned.

The worker and equipment should be kept clean. The worker should wear hair covering and a clean coat or apron over their own clothes. To keep air and dirt off of the meat, the meat should be kept in a clean container with a cover, if possible. As soon as the meat is cut, it should be wrapped, sold fresh, preserved or safely stored to prevent spoilage. When meat is left in temperatures greater than 4 C (40 F) it will begin to spoil after 2 to 4 hours. The meat will not be suitable for humans to eat and can cause illness.

Chapter 23
Beef Carcass Further Processing

Beef Carcass Processing

PHILIPPIANS 4:6

Be anxious for nothing, but in everything by prayer and supplication with thanksgiving let your requests be made known to God.

Two methods of beef carcass processing (cutting) are described. These include: 1—Hot Boning Method and 2—Primal Cut Processing.

1. Hot Boning Method

Hot Boning

1. Hot boning reduces the cost and time to chill out a carcass. The process of slaughter and processing may be done during one work day. Major muscles that may be chilled later for further processing into roasts can be pulled during hot boning.

2. Hot boning is desirable if the carcass will be utilized for sausage or ground products. The carcass will not need to be chilled, but may be boned after thoroughly washing the carcass.

3. The easiest way to bone out a carcass is to keep it hanging and begin boning out the forequarter. Muscles may be boned intact or nearly intact by following the bones.

4. The large shoulder muscle should be the first muscle to be boned from the scapula. The scapula may then be removed and meat removed from around the adjoining bones. This will free the forearm, which can be placed on a table and boned out.

5. The entire rib-eye muscle of the forequarter may be removed by following the vertebra down towards the neck. Remember to remove the neckstrap (*ligamentum nuchae*). Continue removing muscle, leaving the bones as clean as possible without taking excessive fat or cartilage or tendon with the muscle.

6. The hindquarter may be separated into parts. The shortloin or the entire loin may be removed from the round to make it easier to bone-out on a table. The loin is removed with a saw cut below the aitch bone.

7. If no table is available, the loin can be boned by first removing the tenderloin muscle on the underside of the backbone behind the area of the kidneys. Care should be taken not to score (cut deep) the muscle and to remove it in one piece with the fat cover.

8. Next the loin-eye muscle may be removed by following up the backbone upwards. After the loin region has been totally boned, remove the backbone by working a knife around the vertebrae joint next to the sirloin.

9. The sirloin can be more difficult to work with while hanging. If at all possible the sirloin should be removed by making a saw cut below the aitch bone. The sirloin may then be easily boned out on a table.

10. A carcass that is still hanging may be boned out, if the hindquarter is lowered down to a working level for the boner. The sirloin is boned by following the pelvic bone (*ischium*), and sacral vertebra.

11. The round can be boned out as it hangs. The top and bottom round are easily separated following the length of hind bone (femur).

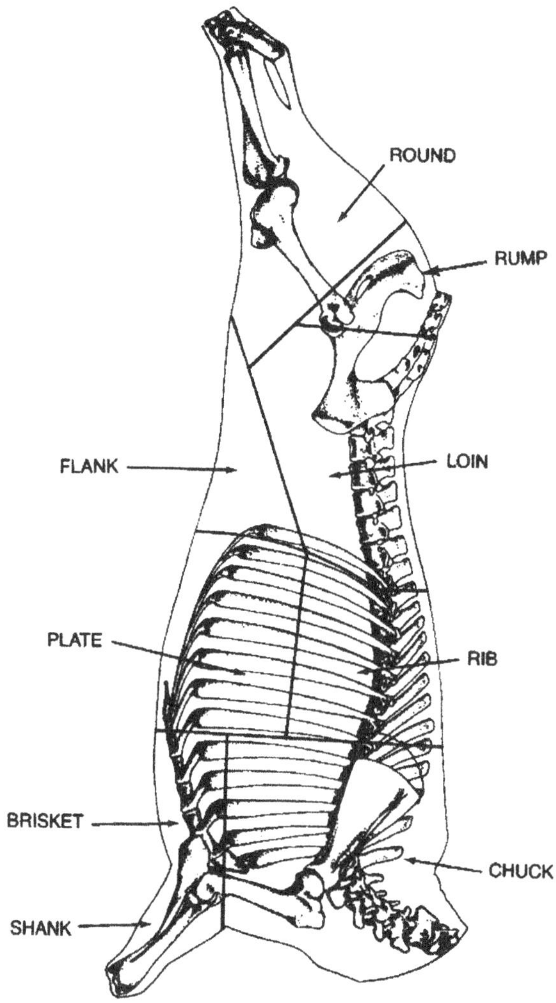

Primal Cuts of Beef.

Beef Carcass Processing

2. Primal Cut Method

Quartering the Carcass

1. The carcass may still be left hanging on the gambrel to begin quartering the carcass (after a carcass is cut in two sides, it can be cut in two again). If quartering on a gambrel, care should be taken that one side does not get the other side off center and the carcass falls to the ground.

2. Quarter the carcass by following the last rib down to the backbone. Saw through the backbone. Then use the knife and make a straight cut across the rib eye muscle (*longissimus dorsi*), separating the forequarter from the hindquarter. The rib eye muscle is the longest muscle in the body and makes very good meat.

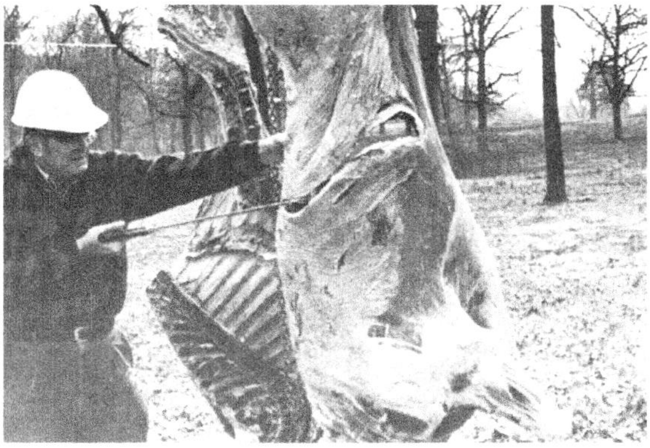

Quartering a Beef at the last rib by cutting through the backbone.

3. Some countries market beef carcasses by cutting between the 12th and 13th rib. Ribs are counted beginning with the first one, closest to the neck area. This exposes the rib eye muscle at its largest size, (and is an indicator for overall muscling). For basic usage, quartering at the last rib will leave all the ribs on the forequarter and make the carcass more manageable in processing.

4. The carcass can then be placed on a table. The table with a washable top that will not splinter when cut is best for sanitation. A long table will be necessary for larger carcasses.

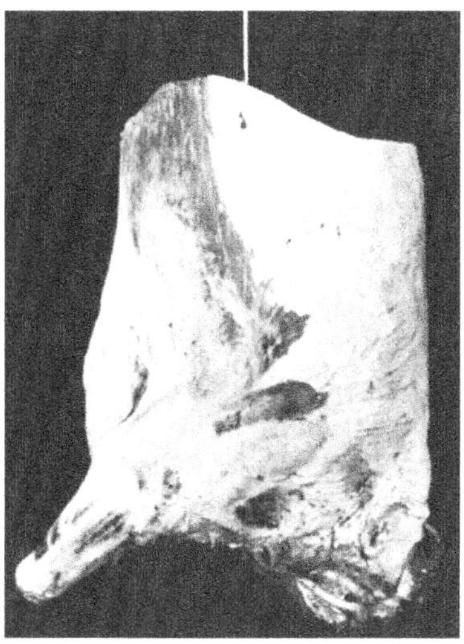

Beef Forequarter.

Forequarter

1. The forequarter is the part of the carcass that has the front leg. The forequarter will be about 52% of the carcass weight and approximately 31% of the live weight.

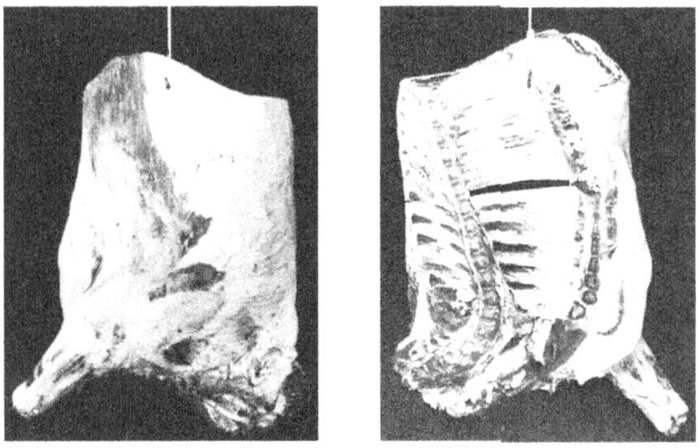

Forequarter and forequarter with knife cut between ribs.

2. The forequarter should be laid on the table with the inside up. Cut with the knife between the fifth and sixth rib or between the sixth and seventh rib, counting from the front near the sternum (bladebone) and upward. The forequarter is turned over and with the saw cut through the thoracic vertebrae and the sternum.

Wholesale Rib

1. With the rib bones facing down on the table, score the top of the rib with a knife approximately 7.5 cm. (3 in.) from the eye on the loin end (small end) and not more than 10 cm. (4 in.) from the eye on the blade end (large end).These measurements may vary with the usage requirement of the rib. On the blade-end of the rib, the blade cartilage may be visible. The rib end can be removed from the plate (full length of ribs) with a saw cut along this knife mark.

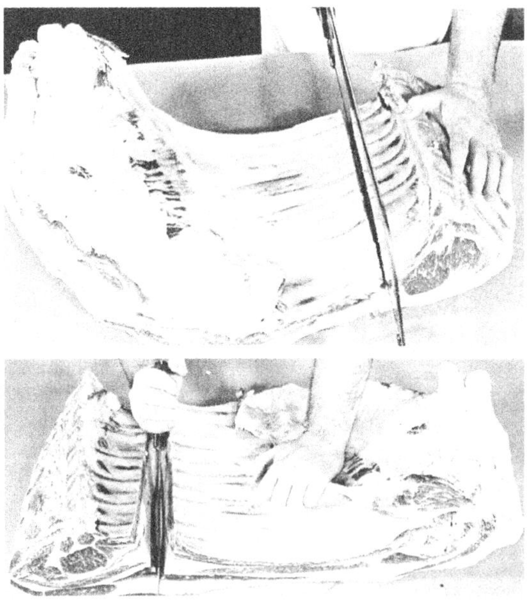

Separating the rib and the plate.

2. The bodies of the vertebrae (chine) bones are removed with the saw to prevent puncturing the packaging material. The blade cartilage may be removed now. To further process the rib, the feather bones (dorsal processes of the thoracic vertebrae) can be removed. This will leave the ribs and the blade bone on the wholesale rib.

3. The wholesale rib may be cut into steaks or several large roasts. After the chine and feather bones are removed, the steaks are easily cut with the knife. The *ligamentum nuchae* (backstrap) is removed. The backstrap is primarily elastin (a hard substance that cannot be chewed or eaten) and will not be palatable (able to eat) when cooked.

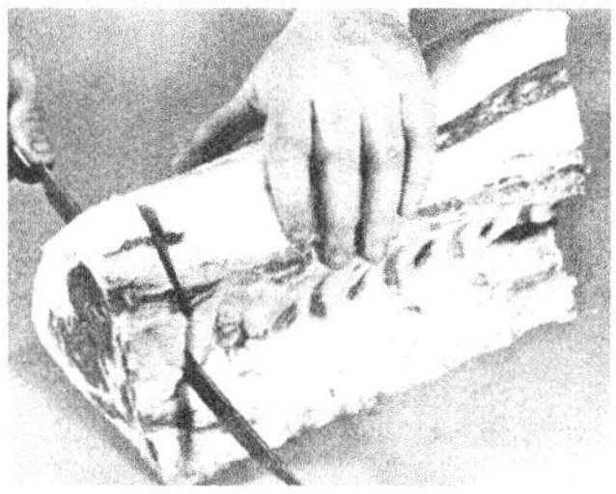

Cutting steaks from rib.

4. Another option to the rib is to remove the cap muscle, which lies over the blade bone. Remove the cap muscle and cut the rib eye roast into steaks and roasts. Any excess fat on the outside of the rib may be removed.

Chuck

1. The chuck is the part of the forequarter that is left after cutting off the rib. The chuck has the forequarter still attached to it. The chuck may be further processed by separating the chuck portion from the brisket and shank by making a cut parallel to the top side of the chuck.

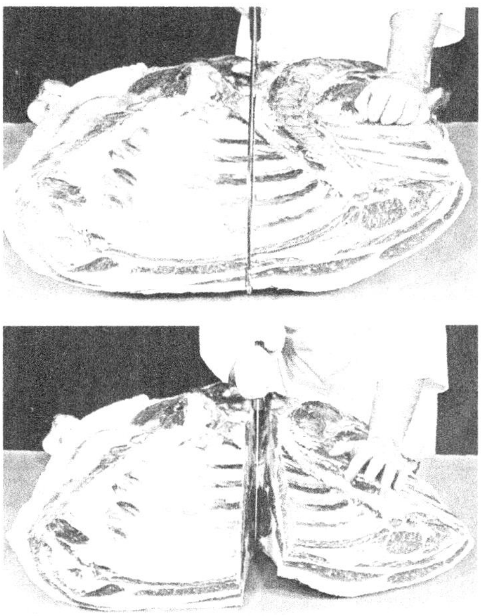

Separating Chuck from Arm/Brisket.

The cut will pass through the cartilage of the first rib and the sternum. This will separate the square cut chuck and make the chuck more manageable to cut into roasts, steaks or to bone out. The thinnest corner of the chuck may be cut off perpendicular to the two cut faces of the chuck to form the cross-rib roast.

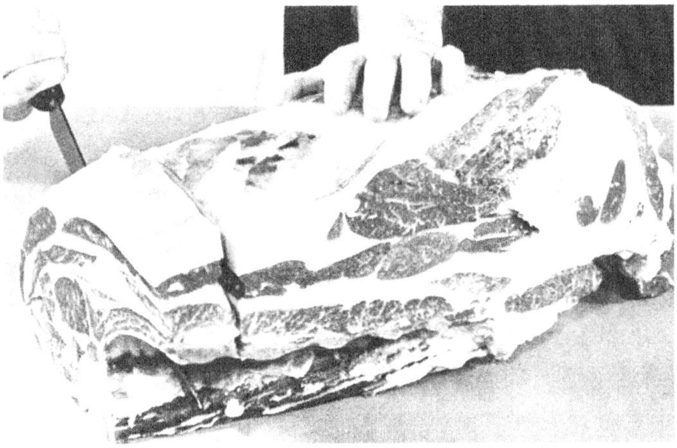

Removing a roast from between the ribs.

A roast is a large piece of meat that is placed in a pot and cooked slowly over a long time to make it tender (easy to chew).

2. The rib and neck bones should be trimmed out from the chuck. Any excess meat can be trimmed from the bones and utilized in ground product. The *ligamentum nuchae* (backstrap or neckstrap) is removed from the chuck.

3. For bone-in cuts the blade end of the chuck may be cut into roasts with a saw. If the roasts are cut approximately 3.8 cm. (1.5 in.), only about three or four roasts can be cut before it goes into the neck region.

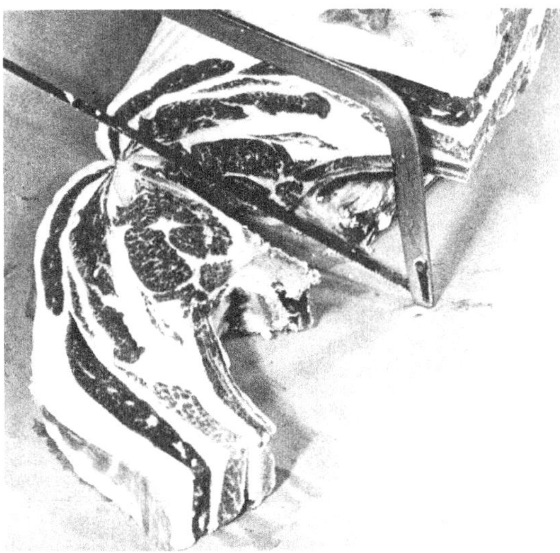

Cutting roasts from rib end.

The chuck should be turned and roasts cut from the arm side of the chuck.

There will be larger muscles on the arm side that will produce meatier roasts. If steaks are desired, the thickness of the cuts can be made smaller.

4. Fat seams should be removed from the bottom of the blade and arm roasts. Any excess meat may be used as stew meat or for ground beef.

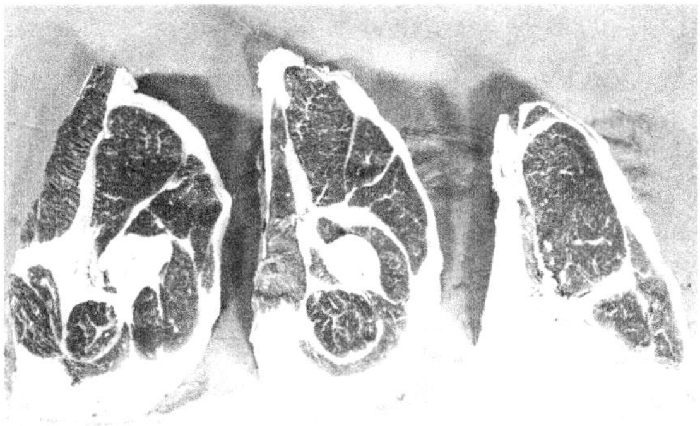

Arm roasts cut from arm end of chuck.

Muscle boning the chuck

1. The chuck can be boned out to produce two large roasts that may be further divided. With the rib side down on the table begin to remove the outside meat.

2. On the arm face follow the humerus (large forearm bone) until it meets the scapula. Follow the spine of the scapula toward the blade face. Do this by moving the blade of the knife down the spine of the scapula (long bone edge that sticks up on the scapula).

3. Continue pulling back the large piece of meat and moving the knife down the scapula. Square this inside roast and trim excess fat as needed. This roast may be tied or netted to keep together for cooking or further cut into two smaller roasts.

4. The *supraspinatus* muscle lies within the scapula and can be pulled out intact for a small roast or steaks. This muscle is also called the fish muscle or the Jewish tender. This is the most tender muscle in the forequarter.

Shank and Brisket

1. The foreshank can be separated from the brisket by a knife cut through the natural seam. The foreshank may be further cut into smaller portions for cooking or boned out for stew or ground beef.

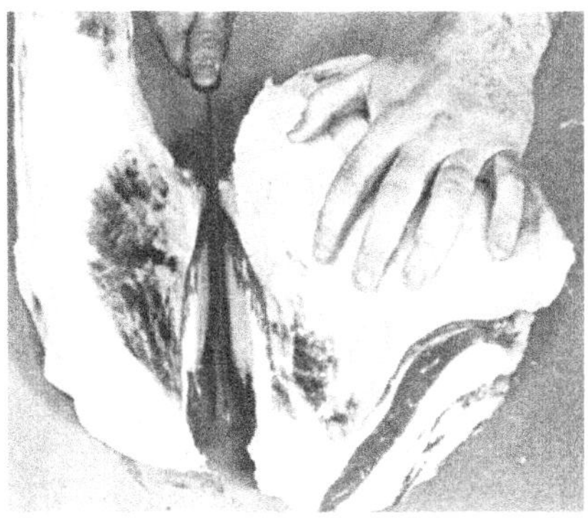

Separating the brisket from the arm.

2. The brisket is the portion of meat that is between the front two legs of a live animal. The brisket should have the flat bone removed and excess fat trimmed to leave a good-sized roast. The brisket may be cut across the middle portion to leave two roasts.

Plate or Short Plate

1. The plate is the section that contains the ribs and can be boned out separating the lean from the ribs and used for stew meat or ground beef. The diaphragm muscle (skirt) separates the thoracic area (area of the lungs and heart) from the abdominal area (area of internal organs). After the membrane covering has been pulled out, this muscle may be removed from the plate and then rolled or kept as thin steaks.

2. If the plate is not boned out short ribs may be cut. To do this, cut the ribs into smaller manageable sizes keeping all the meat and fat on the ribs.

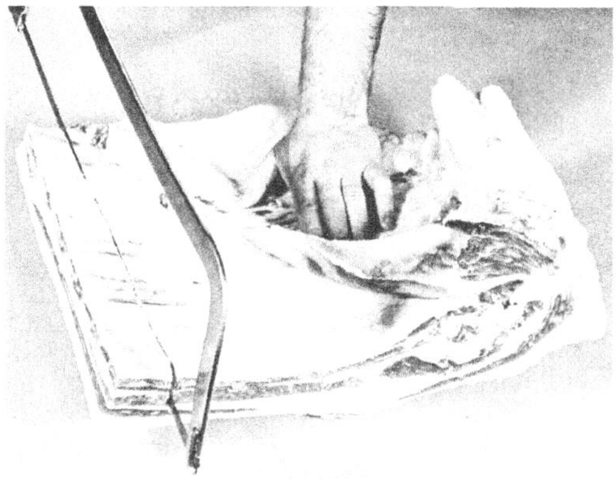

Cutting short ribs from the plate.

Beef Hindquarter

Hindquarter

1. The hindquarter is the back end including the back and the hind legs. The hindquarter composed 48 percent of the carcass weight and 29 percent of the live weight. The hindquarter has the more desirable cuts of meat that are used as roasts and steaks.

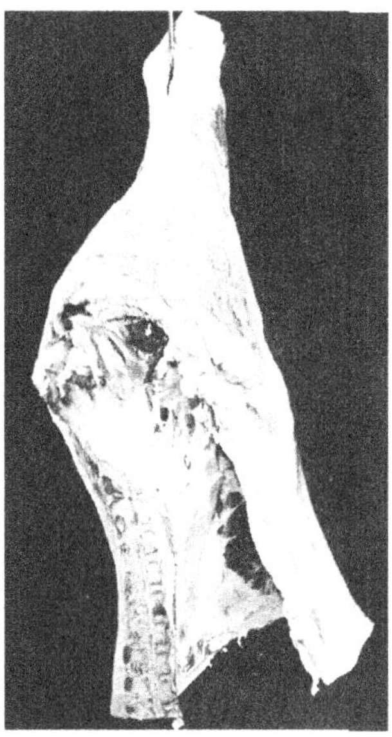

Beef Hindquarter hanging.

Flank

2. The flank is removed by following the contour of the round and removing the cod, or udder fat, with the flank. Cut the flank down to 15 cm. (6 in.) from the loin eye muscle. Care should be taken not to cut too close to the loin eye. After the membranes covering the internal surface of the flank are pulled off, the flank muscle may be removed. One flank muscle will be on each side. This can be used as a rolled roast or ground up.

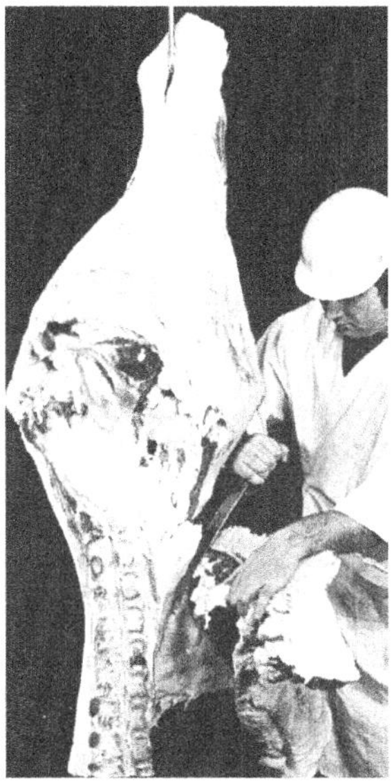

Removing the flank.

Round

1. Separate the round from the loin by a saw cut directly in front of the aitch bone (pelvic bone). This cut is to the rear of the ischium of the pelvic bone and will cut through the bone of the thigh (femur).

2. The round may then be separated into the inside (top) and the outside (bottom) round by following the femur (hind) bone. The outside round is the muscle that lies on the outside of the live animal.

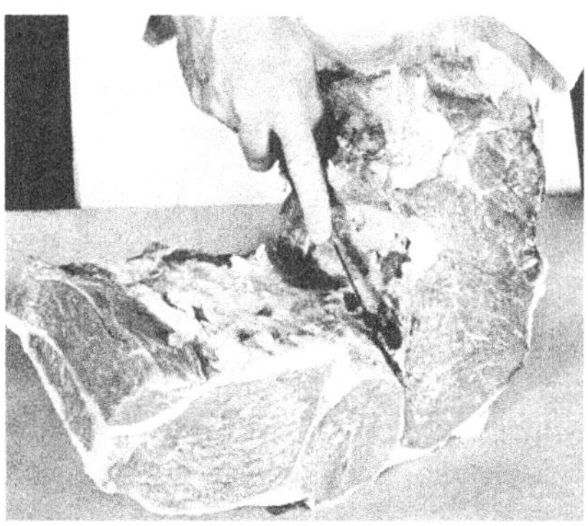

Separating the top and bottom round after removing the femur.

3. The sirloin tip (quadriceps) may be removed by following the natural seam along the femur. Following the femur, the tip will end at the stifle joint at the knee cap (patella).

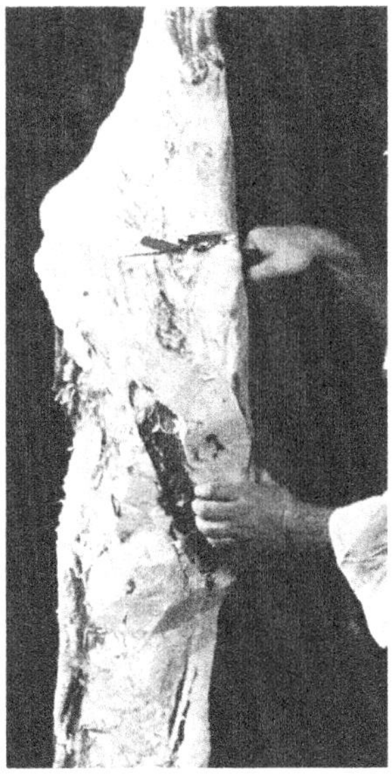

Cutting below the kneecap to remove sirloin tip.

4. The patella may be removed with the sirloin tip, then cut away from the muscle. The outside (cap) muscle can be cut off to remove the excess membranes and fat tissue. The tip is lean and makes a good roast or may be cut into steaks.

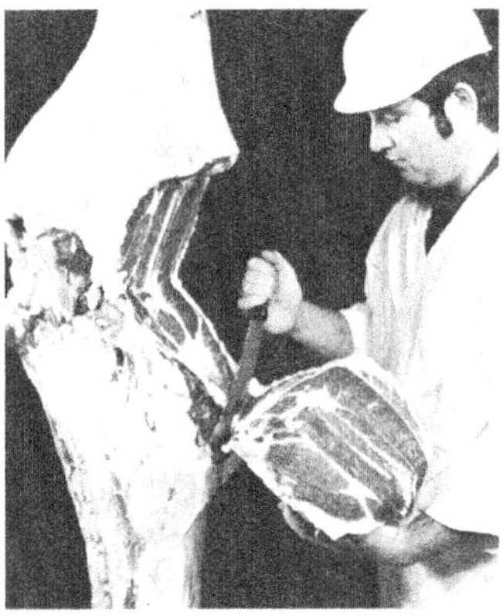

Removing the sirloin tip.

5. After removing the tip, the femur (large hind leg bone) will be exposed on one side of the full bone-in round. Next, the hind shank bone (tibia) should be removed next. The muscles around the tibia should be boned out up to the stifle joint. The joint of the femur and tibia may be disjointed with a knife to remove the shank bone.

6. The femur bone can easily be removed by following the length of the femur with the knife. The outside round may be separated from the inside by following the natural seam that separates them. The top round may be cut into smaller roasts or cut into steaks with the knife. The popliteal lymph node and the surrounding fat should be removed from the bottom round. The heel of the round may be separated from the lower portion of the bottom round. The heel of round is utilized best as a roast with moist heat or ground since it contains a large amount of connective tissue.

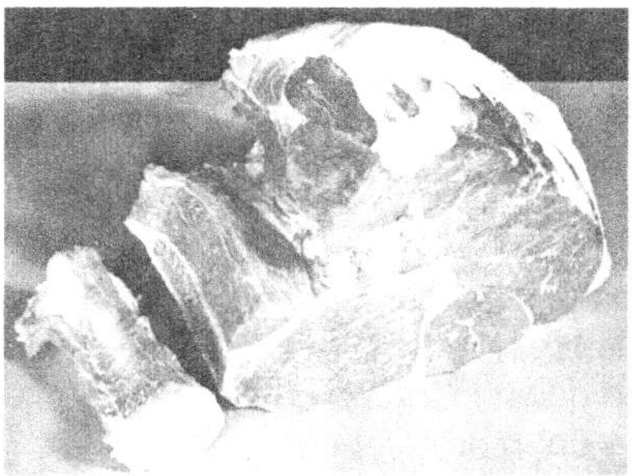

Femur bone removed.

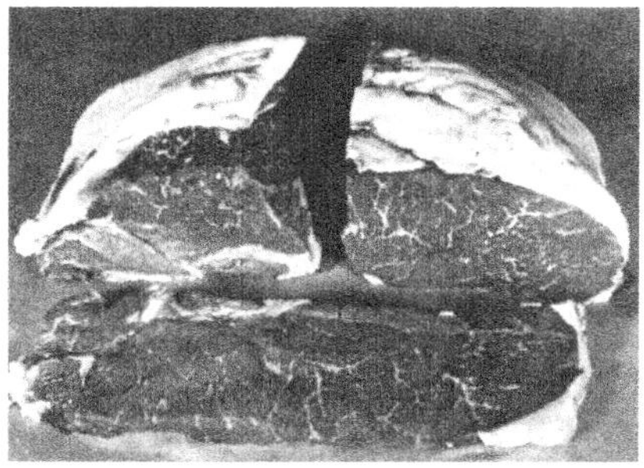

Top round steak and roasts.

7. Using a knife, cut the bottom round into roasts or steaks. The eye of the round is the roundest muscle and should be tenderized. All portions of the bottom round may be tenderized. Tenderizing is done with a knife slightly scoring the muscle, mechanical tenderization or using a hand held tenderizer.

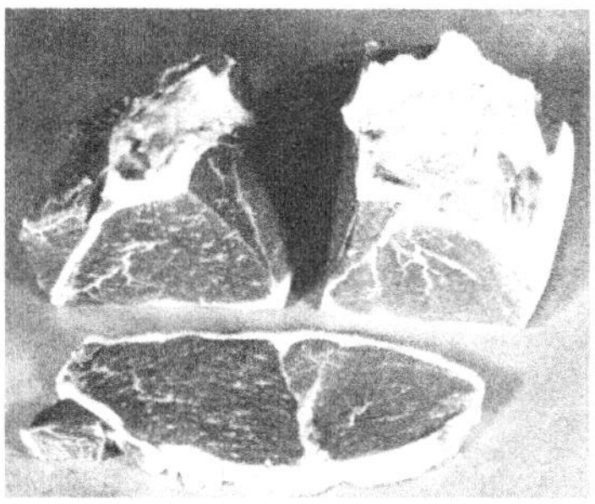

Bottom round steak and roasts.

8. The rump roast is separated from the loin by a saw cut at a point between the fifth sacral vertebra and the first coccygeal vertebra and the anterior tip of the end of the aitch bone. This cut will expose the femur. If a piece of the femur no greater than a silver dollar is cut, it has been cut correctly. The rump roast will still contain the aitch bone. The aitch bone is shallow and may be easily boned out by keeping the knife blade close to the bone.

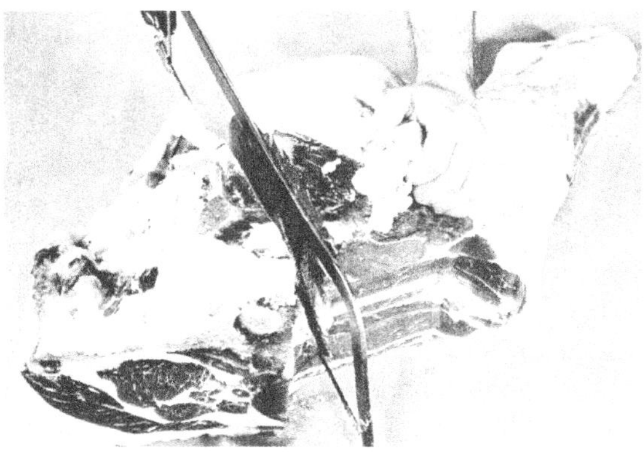

Removing the rump.

Alternate method of separating the round from the loin

1. An alternate method of removing the sirloin tip is with the hindquarter still hanging. Find the knee cap, cut from the stifle joint down the front of the femur. Pull the sirloin tip out and down as the knife separates it from the bone.

2. Next separate the round from the loin with a saw cut between the fifth sacral vertebra and the first caudal vertebra anterior to the aitch-bone. This may be done on a table or even while the hindquarter is still hanging.

Loin

1. In the United States the loin is separated into the sirloin and the shortloin subprimals to market the various types of steaks in each. If an electric saw is available, the entire loin may be cut into steaks beginning with the round end down to the rib end. Steaks can be cut from 2 cm. to 5 cm. (.75 in. to 2 in.) thick dependant upon preferences.

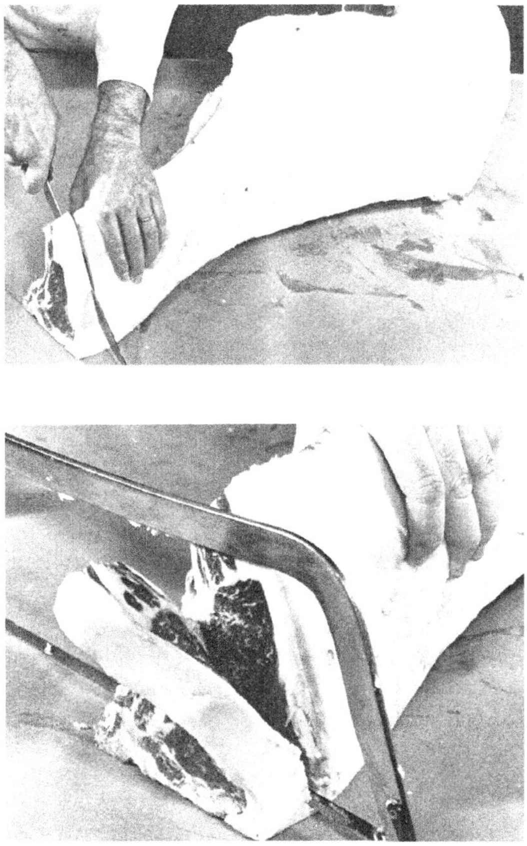

Removing steaks from the loin.

Sirloin End

1. The sirloin end is the end of the loin that is separated from the round. Steaks cut from the sirloin end will have various shapes of bones and will vary in the amount of meat depending upon the location of the cut.

2. The first cut will have a portion of the pelvic bone (ilium) in the shape of a wedge. As the next steak is cut the shape of the ilium becomes rounder. The next few cuts will expose the ilium and the sacroiliac joint leaving two large bones in the steak cut.

3. The hipbone with cartilage will be one of the last cuts made for steaks. After cutting bone-in, the bones may be cut out to leave only the meaty portion of the steaks.

4. Separate the sirloin subprimal from the shortloin with a saw cut between the fifth and sixth lumbar vertebrae.

5. The sirloin may be boned out following the pelvic bone (avoiding cutting into the muscle).

6. After boning out the sirloin, trim any cartilage or membrane. Boneless sirloin roasts may be made from the larger cut or boneless steaks may be cut across the entire sirloin.

Shortloin End

1. The shortloin has the most desirable steaks in the body, so care should be taken not to score the muscle. The shortloin end may be cut as described above with an electric or hand saw into smaller roasts or steaks.

2. The steaks will have predominantly the *longissimus dorsi* and the psoas major (tenderloin muscle) that will be separated by the transverse process (looks like a "T" shape) of the lumbar vertebrae.

3. An alternate method of cutting the entire loin is to remove the tenderloin muscle (most tender muscle in the body). The tenderloin is on the inside of the lumbar vertebrae and runs from the tip in the sirloin to the larger muscled rib end. The muscle must be carefully removed to prevent scoring of the meat. The accessory muscle and the membranous fat layers are removed for a tenderloin which can be cut into filets.

4. The chine bones are trimmed at an angle on shortloin end. The end or tail of the shortloin may be cut within one inch of the loin eye muscle if an electric saw is available. After trimming the steaks are cut bone-in or the entire *longissimus dorsi* muscle is removed and cut into boneless top loin or striploin steaks.

Ground Beef or Stew Meat

1. Any excess lean muscle should be trimmed of excess fat and membrane, and ground with lean from other animals to make ground beef. If the ground beef is going to be utilized immediately the fat from the animal may be used. If the lean will not be used immediately and will be frozen it is advisable not to add the fat until time to be used. And then add fresh fat.

2. Stew meat is cut from larger pieces of lean into approximately 2.5 cm. (1 in) square pieces. These pieces should be trimmed free of fat and membranes. Stew meat can be utilized in more methods than just stew. The size and leanness makes stew meat versatile for many types of meals.

(Photos from USDA 1978)

Chapter 24
Pork Carcass Further Processing

Pork Processing

Psalms 37:25

I have been young, and now I am old. I have not seen the righteous forsaken, or his descendants begging bread.

Chilling of carcasses after slaughter is important not only to reduce microbial counts, but also to firm the fat and muscle. The firmer the fat and muscle, the easier it is to cut.

However, if all the meat is going to be ground up or used for sausage, the meat may be removed from the bone while the carcass is still warm. This should be done quickly after the slaughter process is finished and the carcass has been washed. Remove the meat by following the bones. The carcass may be split in two, to ease in boning out the meat, one side at a time.

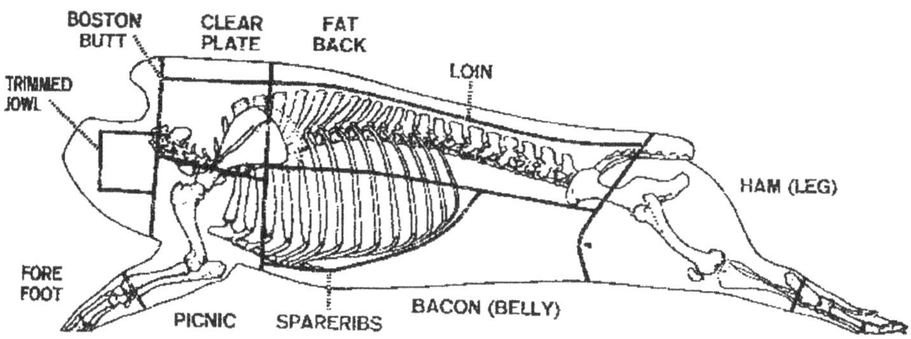

Primal Cuts of Pork.

Pork Processing

Head and Jowl

1. If the head is still on the carcass, remove it by sawing straight down through the first joint on the skull.

2. The jowl is removed by cutting perpendicular to the cut used to remove the head.

Shoulder

1. Remove the shoulder by cutting in a line parallel to the head removal line, between the 2nd and 3rd rib from the front of the carcass.

2. This cut will go through a portion of either the 2nd or 3rd rib and through the thoracic vertebrae.

3. Shoulders have been traditionally separated into the picnic and the (Boston) shoulder. Using a saw, follow the thoracic vertebrae line down the shoulder.

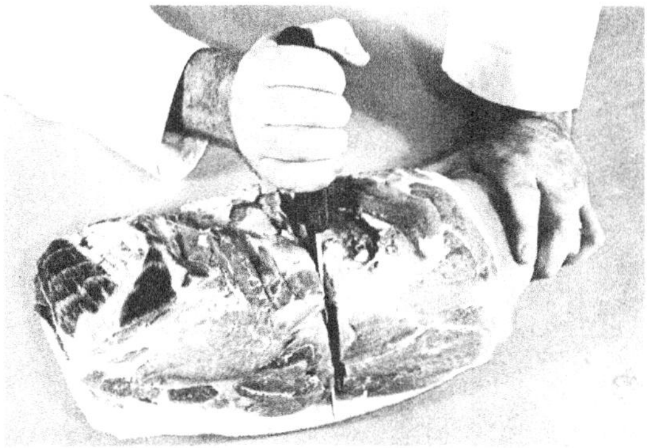

Separating the picnic and Boston shoulder.

4. The picnic will have the foreleg which may be cut off either at the hock or the elbow joint.

5. The removed foreleg can be further smoked or boned out for sausage.

6. The Boston (square cut) shoulder will be squared off after removal from the picnic. The vertebrae can be pulled off the top of the shoulder and then the shoulder cut into steaks (chops).

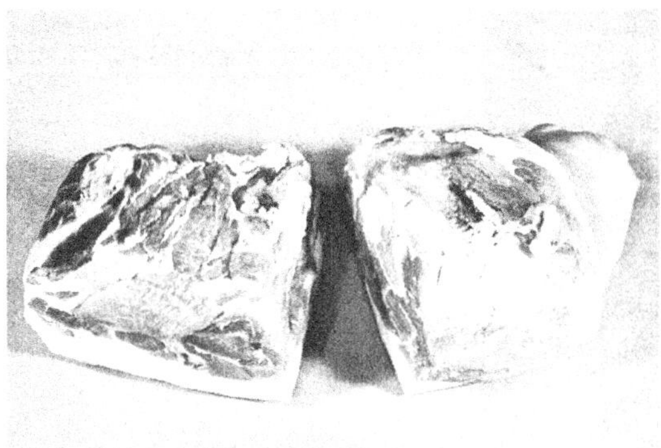

Boston and picnic shoulder.

The steaks may be cut 2.4 cm to 5.0 cm (1 to 2 inches) thick or cut into two smaller roasts. A roast is considered anything cut thicker than 5.0 cm (2 inches).

7. The fat is removed from the back of the shoulder cuts and further processed or can be left on the shoulder.

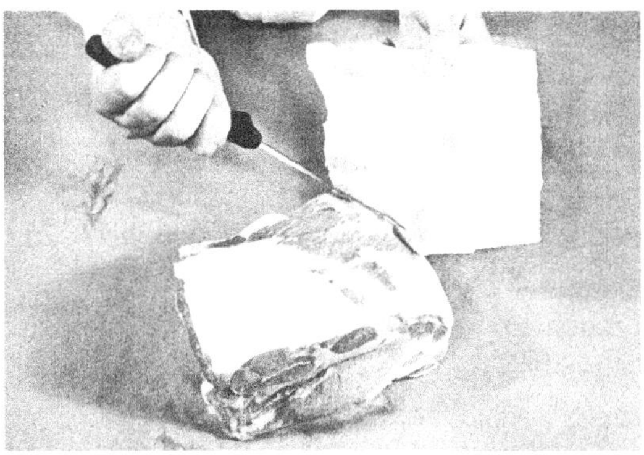

Trimming fat from the Boston shoulder.

The shoulder may be smoked whole. To make a whole shoulder, remove the top vertebrae (do not separate the picnic and the Boston shoulder). Shoulders can be boned out and rolled for roasting.

Ham

1. Towards the rear of the hog, separate the ham from the loin. First remove the hind hock at the joint.

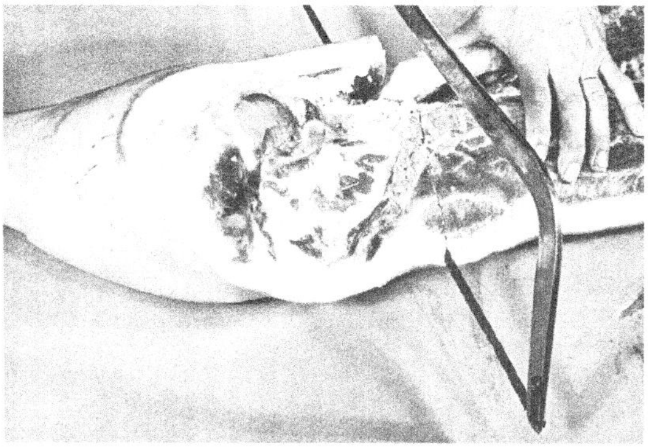

Removing the ham from the loin.

2. Follow the aitch bone and make a cut from the side of the loin at an angle perpendicular to the first cut that removed the hind hock.

3. Trim excess fat off the ham and remove the backbone and the tail.

4. The ham can be used whole (fresh or smoked) or cut into roasts or steaks. The ham may be boned and rolled.

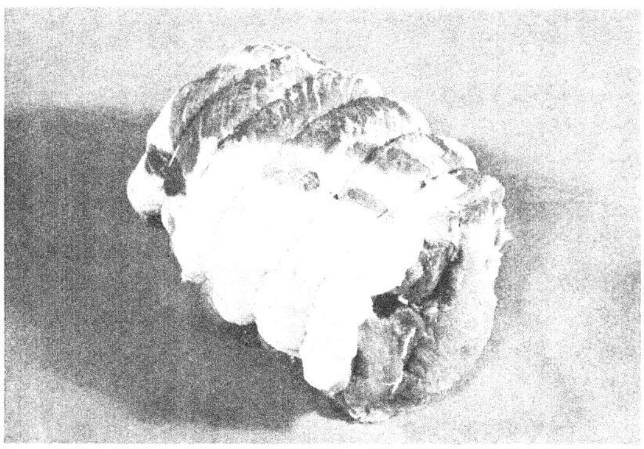

Ham boneless and rolled.

5. The hind hock can be smoked or boned out for sausage.

Loin

1. Separate the side from the loin by following the curve of the backbone. Be careful not to cut too close to the backbone to avoid cutting the rib eye muscle.

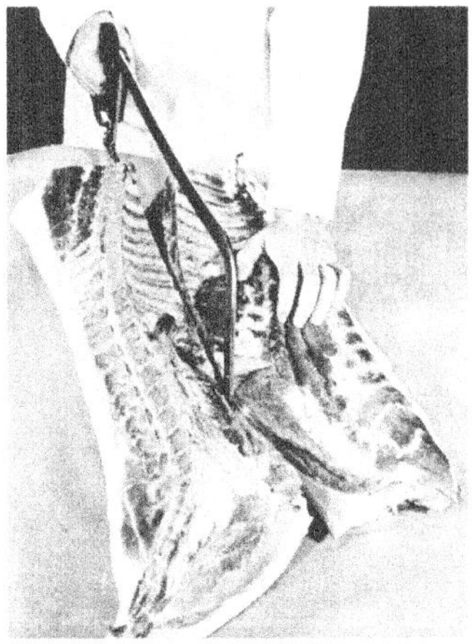

Separating side from loin.

2. Use the knife to cut down from the flank end towards the ribs. Cut through the ribs in a horizontal line through the ribs. This will leave the loin in one piece and the side in one piece.

3. The loin is cut into chops, roasts, or both. The chops may be cut up to 2 inches thick and roasts any size desired.

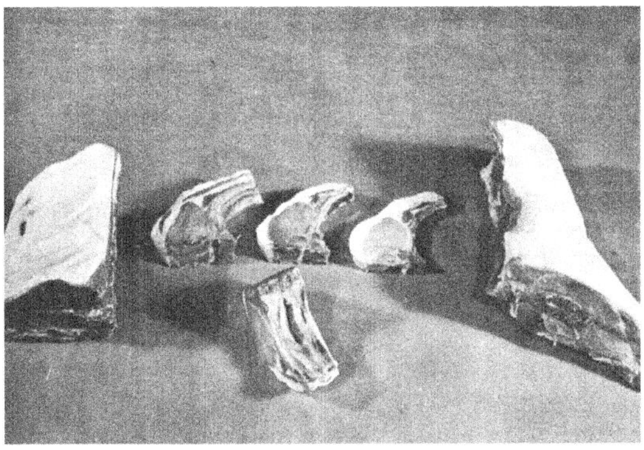

Loin roasts and chops.

4. Excessive fat may be easier to remove with the loin intact than after it is cut into chops and roasts.

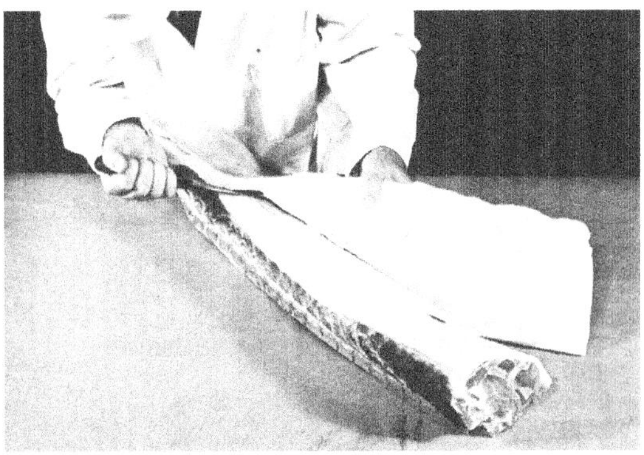

Removing fat from the intact loin.

Spareribs and Side

1. Trim the spareribs from the side keeping the knife flat and moving it up under the ribs until they are loosened.

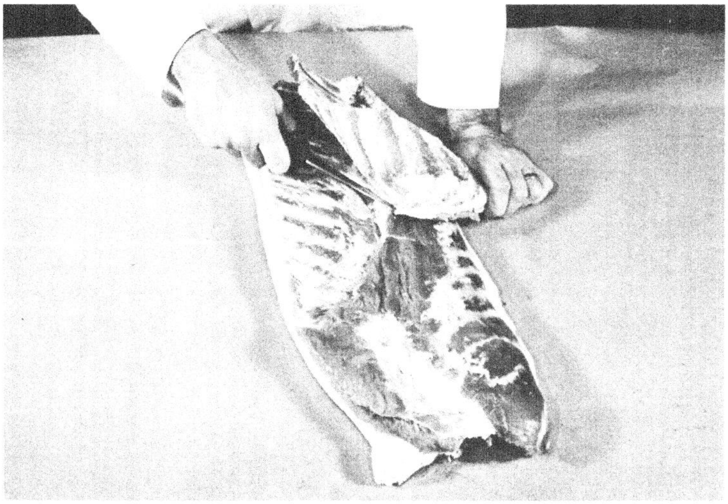

Removing spareribs from the side.

2. Cut a strip off the side to remove the nipples and square up the side. The side is cured and smoked for bacon or kept as a fresh cut.

(Photos from USDA 1978)

Chapter 25

Sheep Carcass Further Processing

Sheep and Small Ruminant Processing

JOHN 1:1-3

In the beginning before all time was the Word (Christ), and the Word was with God, and the Word was God Himself. He was present originally with God. All things were made and came into existence through Him; and without Him was not even one thing made that has come into being. In Him was Life, and the Life was the Light of Men.

Sheep, goats, lambs, antelopes and other small ruminants can be processed and cut up into smaller meat cuts in the same way.

The first step is to remove the thinner cuts of meat from the thicker, meatier cuts of meat.

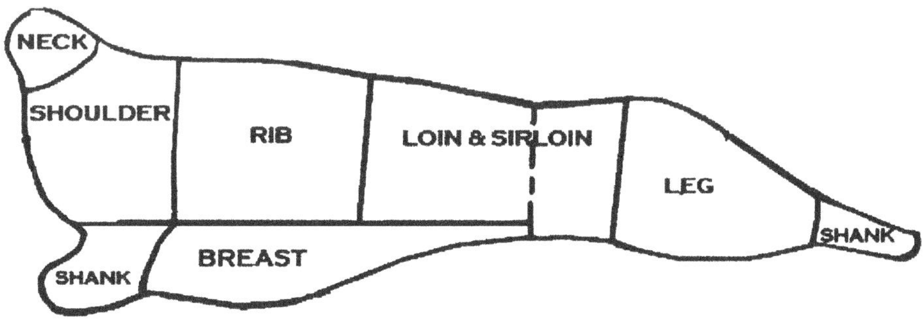

Lamb Primal Cuts.

Remove Flank, Breast and Shank

1. With a single knife cut follow a line from the top where the flank meets the thicker portion of the sirloin down past the ribs, removing the breast with the flank. A saw will need to be used to remove the breast from the ribs and the foreleg from the shoulder.

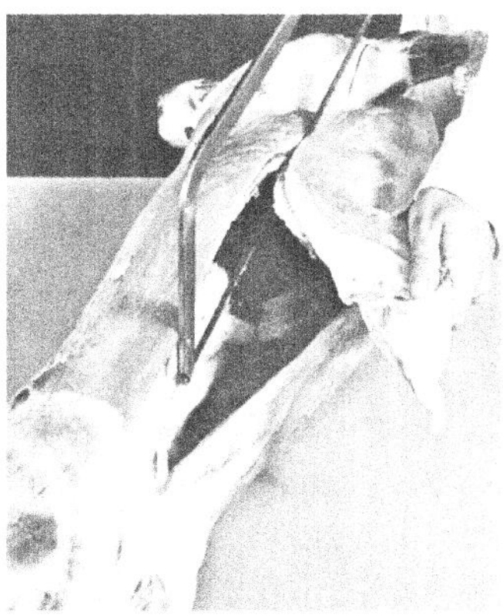

Removing flank, breast and foreshank.

2. The shank (foreleg) is removed by following the line from the breast past where the shoulder and shank meet. A saw may be needed to remove the breast and shank the bone. The flank, breast and shank can be kept bone-in or boneless. If the cuts are boned, they may be rolled and roasted.

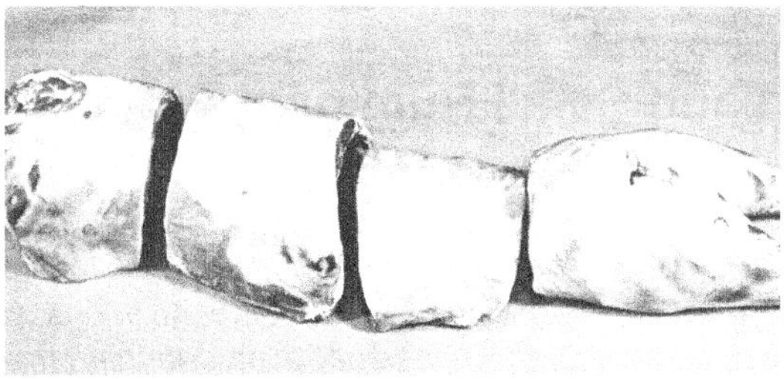

Four primal cuts of lamb: shoulder, rib, loin and leg.

Shoulder

1. A cut made between the 4th and 5th rib will remove the shoulder from the rib portion of the lamb carcass. This cut may be made between any of the lower ribs, depending on how large the shoulder cut is to be made.

2. The shoulder is cut into 2.5 cm thick (1.0 inch) to make chops or steaks.

3. The shoulder can be made boneless by removing the blade bone, top of the leg bone (*humerus*) and also any ribs.

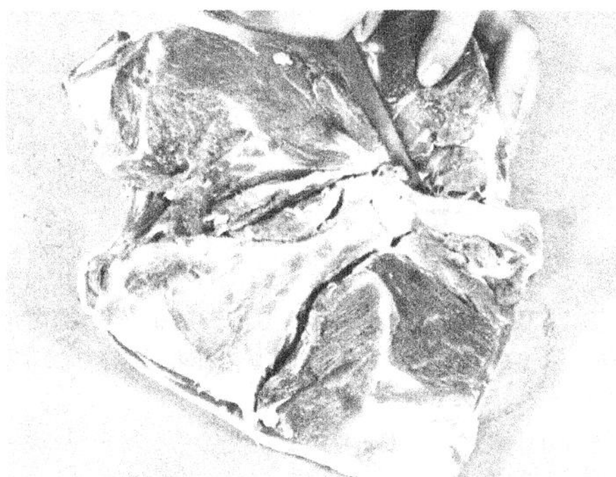

Removing the blade and leg bone from the shoulder.

Rib and Loin

1. If the carcass was left intact at slaughter and not split, it should be split at this point with a saw down the middle of the backbone, making two sides. If the carcass is small, the back may be left in one piece and not cut (split) down the middle of the backbone.

2. The back can be cut at the end of the last rib (12th rib) to separate the rib and loin section. This cut may be made anywhere along the ribs to separate the bonier rib section and the loin.

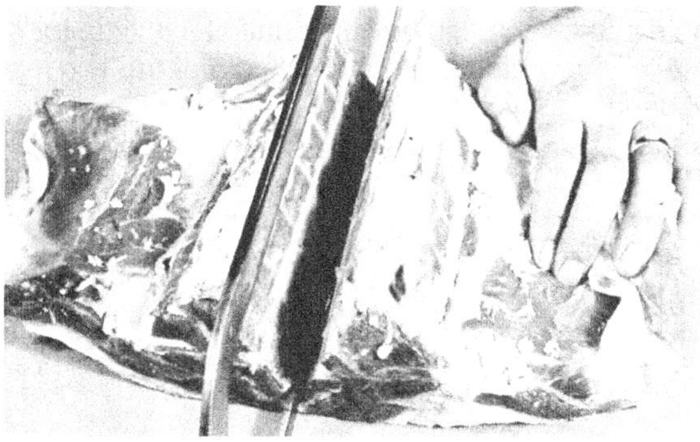

Splitting the loin.

3. The rib and loin once separated can be further cut into smaller cuts of meat for roasting. The rib and loin can also be cut into smaller chops 2.5 cm or less (1 inch or less).

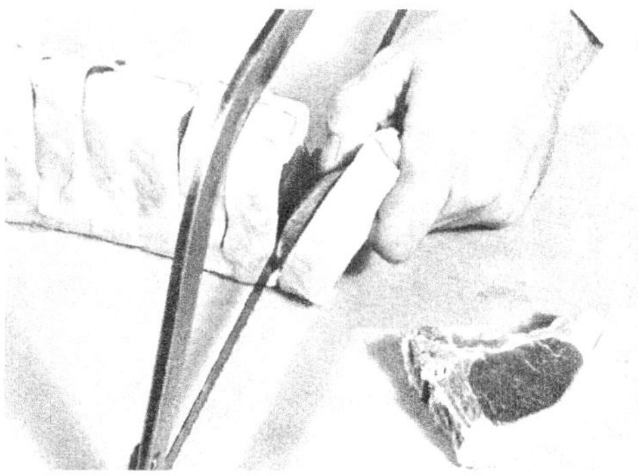

Loin chops being prepared from the loin.

4. The long rib section should be cut with a saw 7.5 cm (3 in.) from the backbone to make a chop with a shorter rib section. The rib and loin can also be boned out for easier storage and cooking.

Sirloin and Leg

1. The sirloin section on a smaller ruminant animal can be left on the leg to make a larger cut of meat. Sirloin chops can be cut off the sirloin still left on the leg.

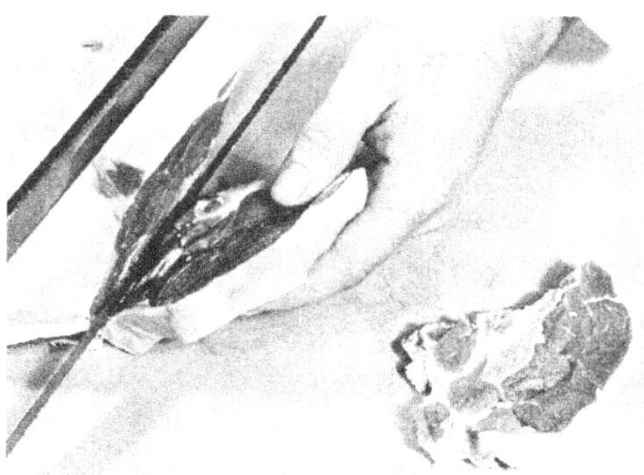

Cutting sirloin chops off of sirloin.

2. The legs of a whole carcass should be cut in half at this time to make it easier to cut into smaller portions. Make a saw cut through the middle of the two legs. This will expose the pelvis bone and tail bone.

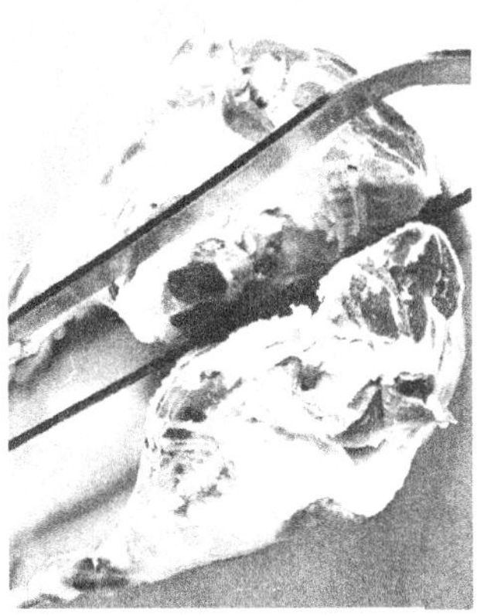

Splitting the legs.

3. The backbone can be cut off of the leg with a knife.

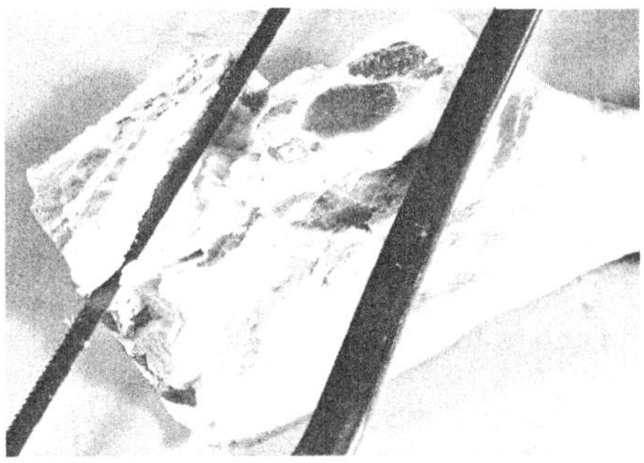

Removing the backbone from the leg.

4. The hock portion of the leg should be removed with a saw; to remove bone from the meatier shank portion. Then remove the shank from the larger section of the leg.

5. The leg should be cut into chops 2.5 cm (1.0 inch) or thinner. The legs may also be boned out and made into a large roasting piece of meat.

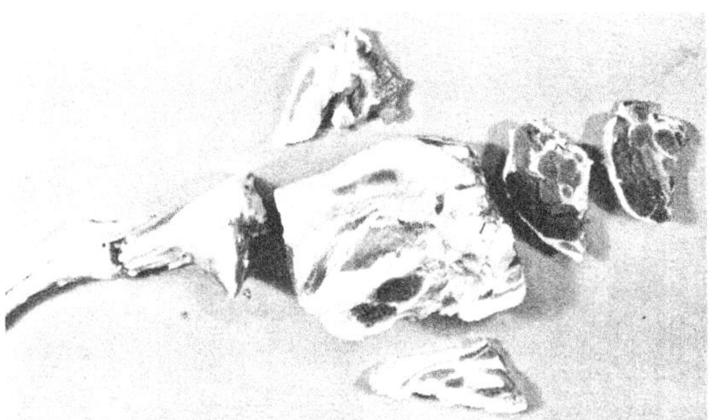

Leg cut into roast and chops.

(Photos from USDA 1977)

Appendix i
References Used

Ashbrook, F. G. 1955. *Butchering, Processing and Preservation of Meat.* Van Nostrand Reinhold Company, pp 73–164. New York.

Atkinson, Dickson, Harbaugh, Law, Lowe, Mohler, Murray, Pearson, Ransom and Trumbower. 1942. *Diseases of Cattle.* US Government Publishing Office. pp 376, 328. Washington DC.

Building Systems of Tulsa. 2003. Gale Plummer, Architect. Tulsa, OK.

FAO Animal Production and Health Paper 119. 2000. Retrieved February 7, 2004 from *http://www.fao.org/docrep/003/t0756e/T0756E00.htm.* FAO. Rome.

Federal Register. Vol. 62., No. 164. Monday, August 24, 1997. Rules and Regulations. USDA/NCDA & CS Facility Guidelines for Meat Processing Plants. Washington DC.

Johnson, E. S. 1986–1994. Meats. Personal Lecture Notes from Meats Course. Goodwell and Stillwater, OK.

Mettler, J. J. 1986. *Basic Butchering of Livestock and Game.* Storey Communications, Inc., pp.124–129. Pownal, VT.

Montgomery, T. M. 1975. Lecture Notes from Meats Course. West Texas State A & M University. Canyon, TX.

Lessons On Meat. National Live Stock and Meat Board, pp 33–49. 1976. Chicago, IL.

Quesenberry, P. and M. Birmingham. 1992. *Where There Is No Animal Doctor.* Christian Veterinary Mission. Seattle, WA.

Romans, J. R., W. J. Costello, C. W. Carlson, M. L. Greaser, K.W. Jones. 1994. *The Meat We Eat.* Interstate Publishers, pp 509–642. Danville, IL.

Tractor Supply Co. 2004. http://www.mytscstore.com.

Turton, Jenny. 2004. *Directorate Communication Parasitic Cysts and Lesions* in Organs. Retrieved February 12, 2004 from National Department of Agriculture. Pretoria, South Africa website: www.nda.agric.za/docs/organs.pdf.

USDA. 1972. *Atlas of Meat Inspection Pathology.* Monlux, W.S., and Monlux, A.W. National Animal Disease Laboratory Ames, Iowa. Veterinary Sciences Research Division. Agricultural Research Service. Agricultural Handbook No. 367. Washington DC.

USDA. 1977. Food Safety Inspection Service. Meat and Poultry Inspection. Training Manual. Washington, DC.

USDA. 1977. *Lamb Slaughtering, Cutting, Preserving, and Cooking on the Farm.* Farmers' Bulletin No. 2264. Washington, DC.

USDA. 1978. *Beef Slaughtering, Cutting, Preserving, and Cooking on the Farm.* Farmers' Bulletin No. 2263. Washington, DC.

USDA. 1978. *Pork Slaughtering, Cutting, Preserving, and Cooking on the Farm.* Farmers' Bulletin No. 2265. Washington, DC.

Appendix ii
Glossary

A

abcesses	rounded area of pus, may have swelling and/ or inflammation around it
abdomen	region of animal that contain the internal organs, the stomach region
abdominal	anything within the region of the abdomen
abdominal	region below ribs which contains the digestive, reproductive and urinary systems of the animal
abscess	rounded area of pus, may have swelling and/ or inflammation around it
actinomycosis	lumpy jaw in cattle, caused by a microorganism, involves the jaw bones and a sow's udders
adhesions	tags of tissue that pulls two surfaces or parts close together that are not normally together
aitch bone	the bone that is found in the hind leg that is part of the pelvis
ante-mortem	before death or slaughter
anterior	towards the front
approved	suitable for human food purposes, passed by health inspector
arthritis	inflammation of a joint and tissue around it

B

backbone	the long bone down the back, made up of many vertebrae (individual bones)
bacon	meat removed from the ribs of a pig, that is left in one piece and cured
bag	udder, mammary gland of a cow
barrow	castrated male pig
bladder	the round sac that contains the urine of the animal, it must not be cut into
blade	the bone in the shoulder that is in a triangle shape and is flat
bone-in	the bone is still attached to the meat
boneless	without the bone
Boston shoulder	name of a cut off the shoulder of a pig that is squared and contains the blade
bottom round	a large roast off of the
bovine	cattle, some buffalo
brisket	the large meat from between the fore legs of cattle
buck	uncastrated male sheep or goat
bull	uncastrated mature male bovine
bung	rectum, anal opening from the intestines that must be tied off to prevent fecal material contaminating the carcass; in the female it also includes the reproduction opening

C

calf	baby cattle or buffalo
cap muscle	the small flat muscle that lies over the rib

cartilage	thin bone-like material found a the end of bones
cervical	neck region
chevon	young goat
chine	the bones that stick up along the backbone
chuck	large meat and bone region of the forequarter containing the fore leg, shoulder and ribs
condemned	animal carcass with a disease or abnormality that makes it unsuitable for human food
contamination	pollution, soiling with infectious or foreighn substance

D

denaturant	substance which will destroy for food purposes any meat or product to which it is applied: changes the appearance, taste or smell so it cannot be used for food
dewlap	region of skin between the front legs of a cow
diaphragm muscle	muscle that separates the thoracic cavity from the abdominal cavity
diffuse	dispersed or spread over a large area
dorsal	towards the back
downer	an animal unable to rise and walk to slaughter
dry landing area	area where an animal will land after it is stunned, must be dry and clean

E

edible	can be used for human food, safe to eat
elastin	stretchy material found in various parts of meat
emaciation	animal that has no flesh, meat or muscle on the bones; bones stick out
esophagus	food tube from mouth to the stomach
evisceration	removing the contents of the abdomen of an animal
ewe	female sheep
extraneous membran	any material on the outside that can contaminate, make dirty: feces, fly droppings, dirt

F

feather	covering of poultry that may be picked off
fecal	droppings from an animal
feces	droppings from an animal
femur	longest leg bone
fetus	unborn, still in the female
flank	inside the back leg
forearm	front arm that attaches to the shoulder
forequarter	front half of a carcass

G

gall bladder	sac that holds the liquid (gall) material from the liver
generalized	spread over, almost all of an entire area or part
grubs	larvae (worms) from the heel fly that will come out of the top of an animal's back and fall to the ground

H

hair sore	sore in beef tongues from licking the hide
heart	surrounded by a membrane and found between the two lungs
heifer	female bovine that has not given birth to a calf
hind bone	rear or back leg bones
hindquarter	back half of a carcass
hip	where the backbone meets the hind legs to form a joint
hipbone	bones that come up from the joint of the hind legs and the backbone
hock	bottom of the hind leg from which to hang the carcass
humerus	bone in the front leg that is the largest and meets the hooves

I

ilium	bone that connects with another bone to form the hip region
incision	cut made with a knife or other sharp tool
inflammation	body reacts to an irritant (something coming into the body), it will be red, swollen, hot and painful
ingesta	food and water taken into the stomach
intestines	long tube of the digestive system that digests food, connects to the stomach and the large intestine
ischium	hip bone, with the ilium forms the hip regioin

J

joint	a bone region where two different bones come together and are held together, so it moves
jowl	meaty portion of the cheek or face of a pig

K

kid	baby goat
kidney	one of two organs found at the backbone of an animal that moves water out of the animal
knocker	person or instrument used to cause an animal to be unconscious before bleeding

L

laceration	jagged tear or wound
lactation	female animal giving milk, udder will leak milk, this is a contaminant on carcasses and must be trimmed off
ligamentum nuchae	long yellow tissue that connects to the base of the head and runs down the backbone, holds the head up
liver	largest organ found inside of an animal that is important to break-down of the animal's food
localized	confined or restricted to a limited area, opposite of generalized
loin	back of an animal, contains the best cuts of meat
longissimus dorsi	the longest muscle in the animal, runs below the backbone
lungs	organs found on either side of the heart, used for breathing, bright pink in color and spongy feeling
lymph node	enlarged area found throughout the body, usually a greyish brown color, will show if any diseases are present in the body

M

mandible	bottom jaw of the head
manure	droppings of an animal
mastitis	inflammation of the mammary gland, udder or milk producing organ
medial	towards the middle of an animal
muscles	makes up the meat of the animal

N

neckstrap	same as ligamentum nuchae
nipples	milk producing glands found on a female animal

O

offal	other parts of a carcass, not the meat, includes organs that may be eaten by humans
orbital	eye socket
ovine	sheep family

P

palpation	physical examination by pressure of the hand or fingers to the surface of an organ or tissue
parturition	act of giving birth
patella	knee cap, covers the joint of the hind leg where the bones meet
pathology	study and determining the disease of an animal
pelt	skin and wool of a sheep
pelvic	bony region through the hip, where the hind legs join the back
pizzle	penis of the male animal
plate	rib portion of a carcass
pluck	heart and lungs removed together from a carcass
poll	top of the head
popliteal lymph node	large lymph node found inside the carcass inside the hind leg
porcine	swine, pig family
posterior	towards the back
post-mortem	after death or slaughter
psoas major	small, tender muscle found on the inside of the backbone

Q

quadriceps	large meat muscles found in front of the hind leg
quartering	separating a carcass that has been split (cut) in two, into two large sections

R

ram	mature, uncastrated male sheep
reactor	animal reacting to a specific test given to it by an animal inspector, indicates that the animal may have a disease
rectum	outer opening of the digestive system where droppings (feces, manure) is dropped
redness	increased blood flow to an area, usually from an infection or inflammation
rib-eye	portion of the longest muscle that follows the backbone, very tender

rigor mortis	stiffening of an animal after death
roast	a large piece of meat
round	large meat portion from the hind leg of an animal
rumen	largest stomach of a ruminant animal
ruminant	an animal with a rumen or large stomach with smaller stomach around it: sheep, goats, cattle, antelope

S

sacral vertebra	vertebra in the backbone that are found towards the pelvic, hip bones
scapula	large triangular shaped bone in the shoulder
seam	membrane or fat region that lies between two muscles, to separate the muscles
shackling	taking a rope or chain around the hind leg of a stunned animal to hoist it up for bleeding and moving
shanks	end of the leg bones after the hooves have been cut off, region to hang the carcass from
shoat	young pig
short ribs	ribs cut across to make shorter; to be easier to cook
shortloin	region of the back muscles (meat) closest to the hip region
sirloin	region of the muscle over the hip region
sirloin tip	meatiest portion of the sirloin
skirt	diaphragm muscle that separates the thoracic and abdominal cavities
sound	animal walks freely without limping or any changes in its movement
sow	female pig that has had piglets
spine	backbone with the vertebrae
spleen	long, flat organ found near the stomach
stag	uncastrated male animal
steak	thin sliced piece of meat
sternum	bone in front of the heart and lungs
stomach	large organ that holds food and water before passing it to other organs
subprimal	large cuts of meat before cut into smaller pieces
supraspinatus	large muscle on top of the scapula (large, flat bone) in the shoulder
swelling	increased blood and flood in tissues, makes a puffy appearance to an area

T

tenderloin	same as psoas major
tendon	a tissue that connects bone to muscle, can be tough
thoracic vertebrae	vertebrae in the backbone that makes up the neck
thorax	region behind the ribs that contains the heart and lungs
tibia	smaller bone in the lower part of the leg
top round	smaller muscle removed from the hind leg, opposite the femur from the bottom round
trachea	wind pipe

U

ulcer	open sore on the skin or mucous membrane, such as seen on beef tongue
unthrifty	animal is not healthy, does not gain weight or muscle

urine — water excretion from an animal, from the urinary system: bladder and kidneys

urogenital — combination of the urinary system coming from the bladder and the female reproductive organs

uterus — female organ that carries the unborn fetus

V

viscera — the internal organs of an animal that may be inspected for any abnormalities

W

weasand — food tube from the mouth to the stomach, esophagus

Appendix iii
Index

The Author

Dr. Sandol Johnson
828.980.4087
sandoljohnson@yahoo.com
sandoljohnson@gmail.com
http://sites.google.com/site/sandoljohnson/

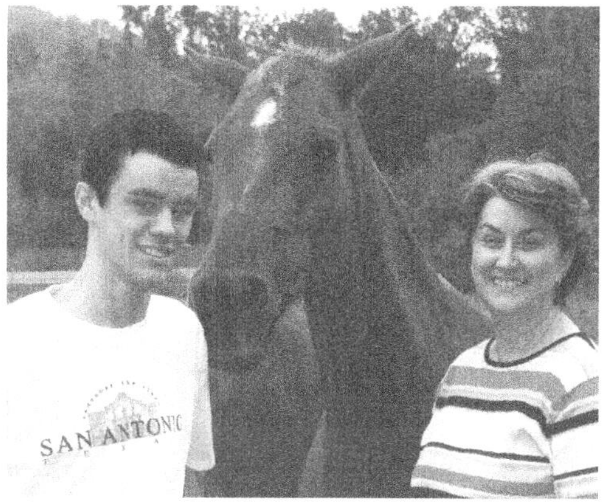

Dr. Sandol Johnson and her son, Micah.

BS	1976	West Texas State University, Canyon, TX
MAg	1983	West Texas State University, Canyon, TX
PhD	1995	Oklahoma State University, Stillwater, OK

Dr. Johnson began her career in meats during her younger years as a 4-H meat judging team member in New Mexico. She continued this interest into her college years as she began to work for the United States Department of Agriculture (USDA), Meat and Poultry Inspection Service. After graduation, she worked for both the USDA's Meat and Poultry Inspection Service and the Meat Grading Service for eight years (1975–1983). During her Masters degree, Dr. Johnson became involved in teaching and managing a meat laboratory for the university. As Associate Professor, she continued teaching and managing the meat laboratory at Oklahoma Panhandle State University for eleven years (1983–1994).

Dr. Johnson has farm slaughtered and processed animals and worked in various countries surveying small slaughter and processing plants. She has traveled in the Caribbean islands, South America, Mexico, and various African and European countries to observe marketing of meat. She has trained individuals and groups in food safety and hygiene, bioterrorism, marketing, zoonotic diseases, and sustainable agriculture.

Dr. Johnson became involved with CVM when her son, then seven years old, signed her up during a CVM display at Oklahoma State University School of Veterinary medicine. She and her son, Micah, work together with a family owned consulting service for small farmers and meat and food processors. Micah has worked in the meat industry and is working on his graduate degree in meat/animal science. Dr. Johnson is the Program Coordinator for the Biotechnology Program at Cleveland Community College in Shelby, North Carolina.

About the Illustrators

Beth Robinson, DVM
14262 FM RD 2073
Vernon, TX 76384
USA

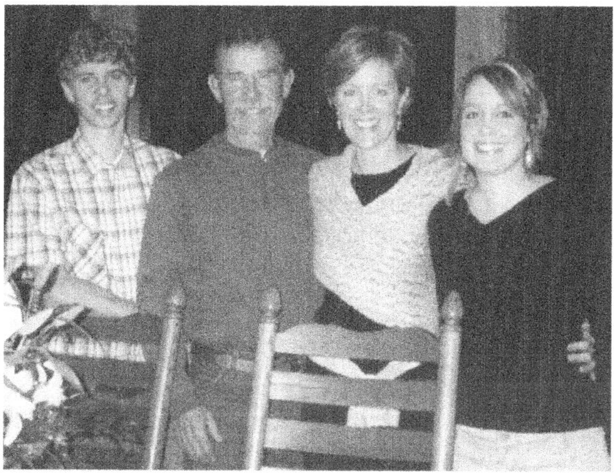

Clay, Don, Beth, Erin Robinson.

B.S.	Animal Science	Louisiana State University, 1979
D.V.M.		Louisiana State University School of Veterinary Medicine, 1990

Dr. Robinson provided the majority of the illustrations within the text. Beth has recently begun relief work again in the Dallas/Ft. Worth area, mainly working on dogs and cats. She began raising Boer goats several years ago to supply her two children with 4-H kids and finds she really enjoys working with them.

She and husband, Don, look forward to his retirement when they can do mission trips and Habitat for Humanity builds.

Todd Cooney, DVM
2132 E 100 North
Kokomo, Indiana 46901
USA
765-452-6051 (work)
765-452-7641 (work fax)
765-452-1831 (home)
cooneydog@juno.com

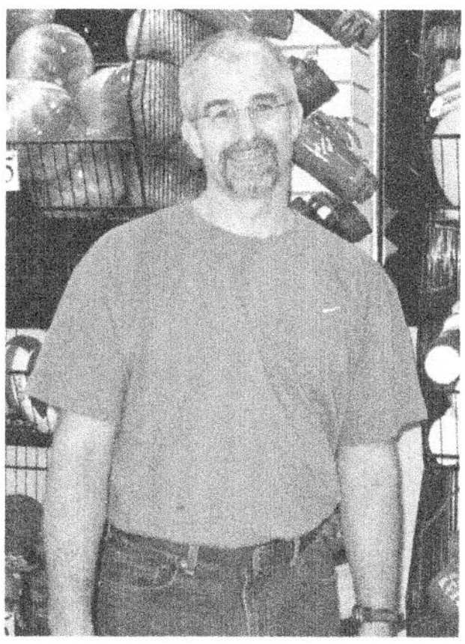

Todd Cooney.

DVM	Purdue University, 1986

Todd enjoys helping CVM by illustrating books and materials. He has always drawn for fun and relaxation, and hopes to glorify God through his artwork. He resides in north central Indiana, has four wonderful children, and feels blessed to be part of the veterinary profession. He is a Purdue graduate, and also holds a master's degree in veterinary parasitology, and bachelor's degree in wildlife science, in addition to Doctor of Veterinary Medicine.

Christian Veterinary Mission (Publisher of this book)

Our vision is to see

Christ's love expressed through veterinary medicine.

Our mission is to

challenge, empower and facilitate veterinarians to serve through their profession, living out their Christian faith.

CVM also provides education and encouragement for those who desire to minister through service, prayer, relationship building, and modeling Christ's love.

About CVM

Christian Veterinary Mission (CVM) is a ministry of CRISTA Ministries, a registered non-profit Christian Service Organization 501(c)(3) based in Seattle, Washington, U.S.A.

CVM was founded in 1976 by Dr. Leroy Dorminy who came to realize the impact that veterinarians could have by integrating their faith with their practice, both locally and around the world. In 2008, CVM had nearly 30 veterinary professionals serving full-time internationally and over 200 veterinary professionals and student volunteers serve on short-term cross-cultural mission trips annually. CVM sponsors fellowship & prayer breakfasts at over 20 U.S. veterinary meetings each year and reaches out to veterinary students through Christian Veterinary Fellowship (CVF) groups in every veterinary school in the U.S. by encouraging them in spiritual growth and professional development.

There are over 3,500 veterinarians affiliated with CVM in the U.S. CVM also partners with organizations and networks in other countries that are focused on empowering Christian veterinarians. CVM has a volunteer advisory board of veterinarians who guide its vision, mission, and programming.

CVM books and the free International Animal Health Newsletter were written with small farmers, veterinarians, and agricultural development workers in mind. Our desire is that they would help individuals and groups develop an appropriate livestock program to meet community needs. CVM's Endowment Fund was started in the early years of the organization's life. The fund provides for meaningful programs that could not be funded by the regular budgeting process.

Made in the USA
Monee, IL
18 October 2026

66036206R10096